All Life Is Yoga

An Exploration of Cosmology and Practice

Mathew Andrews

© Mathew Andrews
matthew@shraddhayoga.org

First Edition, June 2024
Second Edition, October 2024

Title: All Life Is Yoga

ISBN 978-81-975182-7-0 (eBook)
ISBN 978-81-975182-8-7 (Print)

BISAC Code:
HEA025000   HEALTH & FITNESS / Yoga
HEA055000   HEALTH & FITNESS / Mental Health
OCC012000   Body Mind & Spirit/Mysticism
OCC015000   Body Mind & Spirit/New Thought

Thema Subject Category:
QDHC2, Yoga (as a philosophy)
VFMG1, Yoga for exercise
VXA   Mind, body, spirit: thought and practice VXM,
Mind, body, spirit: meditation and visualization V
Health, Relationships and Personal development

Cataloging-in-Publication Data for this title is available from the Library of Congress.

Published by:
PRISMA, an imprint of Digital Media Initiatives
PRISMA, Aurelec/ Prayogshala,
Auroville 605101, Tamil Nadu, India
www.prisma.haus

Contents

What is Yoga? 5
    Auroville 11
    GurujiMa 17
    Arunachala 23

The Evolution of Consciousness
and Planetary Transformation 27

Light and Darkness – Cosmic Forces of Creation 35

Cosmic Forces in Everyday Life 37
    Sūrya: The Sun 41

Yajña – The Vedic Sacrifice 45

The Process of Purification 53

Sādhana – Spiritual Practice and Discipline 67
    Guru: A Guide on the Path 74

Karma, Jñana, and Bhakti 77
    Karma Yoga 78
    Jñana Yoga 80
    Bhakti Yoga 82
    Synthesis 85

All Life Is Yoga: The Path of Karma
and The Path of Dharma 87
    Karma 87
    Dharma 89

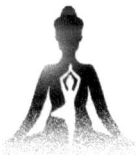

What is Yoga?

Yoga is a stream that flows through the landscape of India's history. It has shaped India's historical terrain and been shaped by it. More recently, the stream of yoga has flowed across the world and into America, though in a form that hardly resembles its source.

Essentially, yoga is a set of practices that supports movement along a path which leads to a state of being. Historically, the word has been used for all three: the practices, the path, and the state. The practices generally involve some type of control, like keeping the body still in a specific position, slowing the pattern of breathing, withdrawing the senses from contact with outward objects, and focusing the mind. They also include things like fasting, cleaning the body, and maintaining integrity in relationships, all of which require controlling our impulses.

The practices of yoga support movement along a path of yoga. This path leads from the experience of separation and isolation to the experience of unity and oneness. It leads from the embodied self feeling like it's an individual entity involved in an existential competition against other individuals for access to scarce resources to the embodied self knowing that it is one with all existence. This is the state of yoga, the union of the embodied self with the Supreme Being.

What is Yoga?

Practices are only truly yoga practices if they support foreword movement along the path of yoga. And a path is only truly a yoga path if it leads toward the state of yoga. Practices found in yoga texts can be done with the intention of enhancing the separative ego: that within us which experiences itself as separate. They can be done to make the body look nice, or to make us more flexible, or to help increase our focus so we can be more successful at work and make more money. None of these things is inherently wrong, but if they inhibit the movement toward union with the Supreme Being, then they are inhibiting yoga.

The modern fitness industry has absorbed a set of practices that were mostly curated by one Indian family and honed them into a product that it calls yoga. This product is wildly popular, and generates billions of dollars a year for those who trade in it. And it legitimately helps people feel better. But whether the people who are selling and buying yoga are actually practicing yoga depends on where the practices are taking them. Are they awakening to the fundamental truth that they are one with all creation and with the Being that breathes the cosmos into existence?

Yoga is not about feeling or getting better, stronger, healthier, or happier. It is not a workout routine or a personal empowerment program. Yoga is union in the most fundamental and comprehensive sense: union of spirit and matter, human and Divine. It is a joining of the mental/emotional personality with the soul, the body with the Earth, the heart's aspirations with the future. It is a cry from the heart of the Earth that seeks to find within itself the heart of heaven.

Yoga asks the essential questions of humanity: who am I? why am I alive? what is going on here? who are these other beings around me? It is a longing and a seeking and a progressive discovery.

The stream of yoga has flowed through the teachings and lives of countless gurus. Some wrote their teachings down, or were written about by their disciples; some just lived and embodied yoga and nourished the aspiring hearts of those who came to learn and grow. Texts have recorded some of these teachings and lives, snapshots of yoga's course through time. These texts hold more than words: they hold vibration, energy, concentrated wisdom in which we can wrap ourselves, immerse and bathe.

They also hold diverse and varied messages and approaches to yoga, some of which directly contradict each other. Some say that a state of oneness and fulfillment is achieved by escaping the material world. They say that the limitations of pain and fear are inherent to living in a body, and that the best way to escape them is to flee the body, overcome its limitations by mastering its urges and impulses. These yogis renounced the world and rejected the trappings of family, commerce and community to seek their transcendent goal in monasteries, caves and jungles. Others have taught that the state of unity that yoga seeks can be found by immersing in the material world and discovering the inherent divinity in every layer of our being and every molecule of matter.

One thing that I've noticed in my study of yogic texts is that engaging with them means engaging with layers of meaning. There are the texts themselves: ancient, written in Sanskrit or Tamil or other derivative languages, relating the experiences of the authors who lived within a particular historical milieu and had unique spiritual experiences. Then there are the commentaries and interpretations of others who have studied the texts. There is a rich tradition of commentaries in India, rooted in an approach to philosophy that's similar to the aspirations of modern physics: they were seeking a Theory of Everything. So texts were analyzed and dissected and ground to a powder to ensure that they accounted for every possible phenomenon, experience and observable situation that could arise in life. The main difference from modern physics is that there was no dogma of materialism: supra-physical phenomena like the power to see the future or be in two places at once or move objects with the mind were often accepted, and thus had to be integrated into the theory.

What is Yoga?

Yoga is an infinitely complex landscape of intersecting lineages, traditions and streams of wisdom. Sometimes these streams crash into each other and create a swirl of conflicting ideas and stories. Sometimes they merge sweetly and harmoniously. What I have written inherently oversimplifies these interactions and relationships, the arguments and collaborations that have taken place over thousands of years. And inevitably I assert my own feelings, ideas and perspectives. In this way I join a long line of commentators who have interpreted and contextualized the writings of yoga for thousands of years and who shared the texts through the prism of their own inner experience.

I am not a technical scholar. My understanding of Sanskrit is limited, and I have a skeptical view of all the historical theories I have come across related to the origins of yoga. What I draw from most is years of seeking the place where spirit and matter mingle. I've attempted to write something that shares more than just information about the history of yoga, something that is relevant to a modern western life. These ancient texts carry a depth of practical wisdom that offers us new ways of understanding our present milieu. I've tried to bring some of that wisdom into expression.

The modern capitalist yoga culture manipulates the mystique of yoga to engage consumers and sell products. Many modern yoga teachers and businesses, some with a superficial understanding of yoga and little expression of honor or gratitude to the Indian culture that produced it, have used the aura of an ancient mystical science that promises liberation from suffering to profit themselves at the expense of others. So while maintaining humility and reverence for the teachings themselves, we can leverage the deepening of discernment that yoga offers to thread the needle between the hubris of modern 'science' and the rampant cultural appropriation of modern yoga culture.

This includes your engagement with this book, dear reader. I have spent decades studying yoga and traveling back and forth from India, compelled by a love for yoga that even I don't fully understand. All I can offer you is my own lens, my own heart, my learnings and perspectives. This book is an offering at the feet of Ādiyogeshvara, the Lord of Yoga. I pray that it serve the purposes of awakening and freedom from suffering that yoga has served for thousands of years, and I ask that you forgive the places where my ego asserts itself and obscures the truth.

My seeking and understanding of yoga has been shaped by many teachers, texts and experiences. But three stand out among the rest, and these three form the foundation of what I will share in these pages. The first influence is the Mother and Sri Aurobindo, whose influence and teachings I have absorbed through their recorded words and the communities and spaces that they inspired. The Mother and Sri Aurobindo taught an Integral Yoga that sought to reconcile and synthesize the divisive arguments that have defined various yoga schools throughout history. They looked for the essence of each approach, and noted that it's in a path's rigidity and rejection of other paths that falsehood dwells. Each true path of yoga leads to the same destination and has the same aspiration at its root, and by seeking that commonality we can use any approach with sincerity as supports for our journey of self discovery.

They described a yoga of the Earth, a great collective awakening that includes every person, every animal, every microbe, even the living Earth Herself. Their yoga was an integral commitment to realize our union with God in whatever unique life circumstances we might find ourselves in, and to radiate that realization into the world around us. They honored the path of renunciation, releasing attachment to desire and possession and identity, and taught that it can be integrated into any life, whether in a jungle or in a city.

This yoga appealed to me from when I first encountered it in 2000. It lit the flame of aspiration in my heart and has nourished that flame for decades. And it's Sri Aurobindo's yogic framework that will give shape to and transmit the teachings that we will share with you throughout this book.

My second major influence is GurujiMa, at whose feet I have learned through direct transmission since 2002. She is a living embodiment of the principles of yoga that I have read about in dozens of historical texts. I constantly find that to be with her is to be in the presence of the teachings. Her practical spiritual outlook aligns with that of the Mother and Sri Aurobindo, and she considers herself as serving the same purpose that they served. Her life is entirely offered in service to the Supreme Being, and I experience the energetic essence of the Supreme Being, the great love that holds together galaxies and human communities, as emanating from her.

The third influence is Arunachala Siva, the mountain that wordlessly radiates love and holiness, attracting millions of pilgrims each year as it has for millennia. Arunachala does not speak or write or move. And though it is made of earth and stone, it somehow shines like a sun. The energy that I feel coming from Arunachala is the same divine energy that I feel in Sri Aurobindo's writing, or in GurujiMa's body. It is an energy of holy love and sacred wisdom that transcends beliefs, ideas, or platforms. It desires to help us awaken to the truth of ourselves, the deeper being that animates us and shines through the filter of personality.

These three influences have their own nuances, but there is a core cosmological and philosophical framework that underlies them. And that framework will shape the teachings in this book. I will introduce the basic elements of this teaching framework through the following topics:

> The Evolution of Consciousness and Planetary Transformation
> Light and Darkness - Cosmic Forces
> Yajña - The Vedic Sacrifice
> The Process of Purification
> Sādhana - Spiritual Practice and Discipline

Karma, Jñana, and Bhakti
All Life Is Yoga - The Path of Karma and the Path of Dharma

This book includes a chapter on each of these topics. It is an attempt to articulate my understanding of yoga that has been fostered through deep, consistent immersion in the streams of wisdom coming from these three sources, fused with my study of many texts from the yoga tradition and fascination with the Sanskrit language.

Lert's begin with a few autobiographical anecdotes that can help contextualize my relationship with the three main influences I mentioned above. I'll share how they entered my life and my heart.

Auroville

On my 21st birthday, I stepped off a plane and into a sea of South Indian humidity. The acrid smell of burning trash swirled around me, mingling with shouts from luggage handlers and taxi drivers. The air was sweating, a sharp contrast to the dry bubble of airplane air I'd been wrapped in for what felt like years. I got on a bus and headed south out of the city, past metal-roofed huts and palm trees, packs of stray dogs tussling on the roadside.

I'd come as part of a semester program designed to explore intentional communities. We studied things like governance systems, economic models, whole systems agriculture, waste management, and alternative power sources like wind, biogas and solar. Arriving after 10 days spent in the cloistered and stoic atmosphere of a Buddhist monastery in the south of France, the circus of sights, smells and sounds was overwhelming and invigorating. I unconsciously alternated between bracing myself and inhaling deep draughts of the frenetic, swirling energy.

And somehow, in this most exotic place, I felt absolutely at home. It was as if I'd spent my entire life in a foreign country, and I was finally back where I belonged. The bus's devastated suspension system skipped and hopped over the cracked and pitted road, the guileless eyes of children widened when they saw my white face and long hair, and cows chewed burnt garbage on the side of the road. Families zoomed past the bus, crowded on motorcycles as if they were station wagons. One two-wheeler had a crate full of chickens on the back; a backseat rider on another held a massive wooden door. Heaps of coconuts, strategically positioned at key road junctions, punctuated total chaos and disorder. It all felt simultaneously so alien and so comforting. My senses were overwhelmed and my heart was cradled in an experience of safety and peace.

I felt more at home in this distant, foreign place than I ever had in my life. And it's not that I'd felt especially alienated or alone before. I grew up in a loving home and had lots of friends as a kid. But it was like a veil had been removed, revealing a sense of belonging that I hadn't known was possible. The foreign sights and sounds and smells were strangely familiar, like a forgotten lullaby that reminded me of a time that memory could not reach. I almost felt like I could start speaking Tamil, if only I could breach the barrier of memory and reach far enough back into my past. I felt held by the Earth and at home in my body, comfortable in my skin. India welcomed me with a sweet, loving embrace.

I felt content, safe, and seen by India. The Earth, the air and trees and water felt intimate, and I felt that they recognized me, like I was an estranged family member returning after years away. I opened myself to this strange familiarity. I don't know why, perhaps because everything was so new, but instead of analyzing this experience of comfort and familiarity skeptically and deciding it was incredible, I allowed it to speak to me. I listened with an open mind and an open heart. My openness created space for the experience to expand and deepen.

We drove south along the Coromandel Coast, its name possibly derived from a Portuguese approximation of Cholamandalam, or realm of the

Cholas. The Chola Dynasty lasted at least 1,000 years from 300 BCE to 1300 CE, making it one of the longest-lived dynasties in history. They built incredible temple complexes, intricately carved stone shrines and reliefs, and supported poets and musicians. Sangam poetry, the collection of Tamil compositions from the Chola period, is an enormous wealth of gorgeous verses honoring the natural world, the intimacy of lovers, and the ardor of spiritual devotion.

Small huts roofed with palm fronds lined the road, the outlying homes of villages that retain the customs and traditions of ancient India. Farmers coaxed water buffalo through flooded fields, speaking to them in a language that's been used in these villages for millennia. The bus stopped as goatherds chased their flocks across the road and down bucolic dirt paths toward fresh pastures. There was a rich and expansive history lingering there, a palpable feeling of continuity stretching back beyond writing and record. Fishing boats coasted down lagoons toward the Bay of Bengal, and pools of salt water evaporated under the noon sun in open square pans the size of a suburban yard, leaving behind sparkling white crystals with transformative power.

After three hours of driving, we spotted white sands bordered by the endless blue of the ocean, and then made a sharp right turn up a slight rise toward Auroville. This is the community that we'd come to study, the largest intentional community in the world, where thousands of people have come from dozens of different countries to try building a spiritual city that manifests human unity. When Auroville was founded three decades before my arrival, the land was a moonscape, a red desert where monsoon rains regularly washed the topsoil down canyons and gullies and into the ocean.

By the time our bus jostled and grunted its way up the hill toward the nascent city, Aurovilians had planted millions of trees, reintroducing the native tropical dry evergreen forest that had been decimated by the European timber industry. Stretches of red Earth gradually gave way to young forests filled with shouting birds, mongooses, lizards and snakes. Once, when I had been in Auroville for a few weeks, I stopped my bike in a forest clearing to orient myself, and startled a giant sand boa, thick as my arm. Another time a cobra took up residence right outside the kitchen, wrapped around itself like a labyrinth.

Cycle paths criss-crossed the roads and cows wandered anywhere that wasn't fenced. People with all gradations of skin tone and various accents sped down dirt roads on motorcycles and ate together at outdoor cafes. They had been drawn from around the world and left the comfort of their home countries, where a smile and a nod were immediately understood, and where their dialect was never met with a confused stare. They came inspired by the dream of human unity, Earth stewardship, service to the Divine, and worked alongside native Tamils whose ancestry was older than the villages themselves. The living forest around me spoke of hope and possibility.

Auroville was conceived and founded by Mirra Alfassa, known as The Mother, who collaborated with Sri Aurobindo, an eminent scholar, Indian revolutionary and yogi. The Sri Aurobindo Ashram in Pondicherry developed during the 1920s, 30s and 40s as a kind of laboratory of evolution, a place where Sri Aurobindo and the Mother worked together to foster the future of the human species, which they said was an intermediate phase, a stepping stone between the animal and the Divine Being whose advent is the Earth's cosmic purpose. They connected the ancient teachings of yoga with present socio-political circumstances, and drew a line into tomorrow.

I've always been kind of a dreamer. I was editor of our high school literary magazine, and would stay up all night on mushrooms writing poetry. I have always believed that there is more to life than what we can see and touch. But I'm also very sensitive to the accusation of naivete. I don't want people to think of me as starry eyed or airy-fairy. So I end up looking for the place where spirituality becomes grounded and practical. That's part of what drew me to Sri Aurobindo's philosophy. He was a political activist, a committed agnostic-atheist and practical intellectual. And then he discovered yoga, and he brought all the same rigor and incisiveness to his exploration of yoga that he'd brought to his scholarly and political work. His spiritual teachings stretch out into the furthest reaches of the cosmos and beyond, but they are always rooted in reason. They make sense.

I've had many transcendental experiences, moments where the isolated bubble of self opens and I feel myself joining with the cosmos. If I deny these experiences or call them illusions, I'm erasing a part of my life, allowing the dogma of materialism to override my actual observations. I have felt the soul of the sun just like I can feel its warmth and see by its light. Sri Aurobindo's teachings are like this. They are rational, logical, with one coherent idea leading to another in a clear stream from here to eternity. They remain practical even as they embrace and include realities that science has yet to acknowledge or allow.

Auroville was built on these practical spiritual teachings. It was conceived as a place where spirit and matter could join. If the Sri Aurobindo Ashram was a laboratory of human evolution, a place with rigid rules and boundaries that created a container for experiments in consciousness, Auroville was the field study. It was what happens when you remove the limitations of the lab and take the experiment into the messy and complicated world. I loved it.

Auroville's founding charter states that "Auroville belongs to nobody in particular. Auroville belongs to humanity as a whole. But to live in Auroville one must be a willing servitor of the Divine Consciousness." And right in the geographic center, next to a majestic banyan tree, is the Matrimandir, the soul of the city. Matrimandir means roughly "Mother's temple", and it's a giant golden sphere, like the golden egg of yogic lore called Hiranyagarbha, out of which all creation emerges. It symbolizes the possibility, or as Sri Aurobindo would say, the inevitability, of matter and spirit joining to create a Divine Life on Earth.

When I arrived in Auroville, the Matrimandir had been under construction for thirty years. But in its incomplete state, I could already feel what it would eventually become. I walked in awe through the vast Park of Unity, where people sat silently or whispered to each other, a place suffused with peace and tranquility. Approaching the Matrimandir, I first walked down a path between two tall earthen walls, descending beneath the ground before climbing a marble staircase toward a door in the giant gold sphere.

A narrow opening led to a spiral staircase, and at the top I found myself in a vast central chamber. A much wider spiral ramp hovered in mid-air like a magic carpet. As I walked slowly upward, a slight breeze blew through unpaneled walls, and my heart climbed. A simple joy grew within me that had no context, no story. I felt like I could cry out, dance, hug someone for no reason at all. I wasn't happy about something, and it wasn't anticipation. It was more like joy was the most natural thing to feel, a baseline state of existence, unadorned, needing no support or reason. Joy was the source of my being, and everything that had previously stood in the way, preventing me from experiencing it, had fallen away. Inside the inner chamber, everything was white: the floor, the walls, the cushions and chairs, and the twelve pillars that stood like sentinels around the middle of the room.

In the center, the largest optically-perfect glass crystal in the world caught sun rays that were channeled down through the roof using mirrors. I sat, closed my eyes, and basked in the silence that permeated the space. When I eventually rose and left, that silence stayed with me, resonating inside my heart and around my body. It was not a blank or empty silence, but full, vibrant, holy. In the silence I could feel a pull within me to open myself more fully, a longing to live a life entirely aligned with love and truth. I aspired to stop grasping for control, manipulating people to get what I wanted, and to trust the innate goodness of life. I came to understand this aspiration as the primary vehicle of yoga.

Aurovilians talked about yoga all the time. They considered planting trees yoga, or teaching children, or preparing food, or weeding the garden. Everything they did with intention and for the good of the community, everything that aligned with their life's purpose and supported a more peaceful and harmonious future was yoga. Yoga was anything that helped join the deeper self with the personality, anything that infused the spiritual being into the mental/material being. Sri Aurobindo said "All life is yoga". Aurovilians created their lives and their community in the aura of this statement, open to being shown the path as they walked it, open to guidance and direction from within and without.

Auroville was created as a place to join spirit and matter, human and Divine. It is a place of experimentation, of learning and seeking progress from our current limited human state toward a full embodiment of our spiritual being. Instead of worshiping God on certain days of the week or specific holidays, worship becomes a way of life, interwoven into work, play, self-care, giving, receiving, relating to each other. Auroville represents the promise, not of eternal life in a distant heaven, but of a Divine life on Earth. An aspiration was kindled in me during my time there, and a sense that, despite its limitations, just the fact that it existed was a gift to the Earth. I felt that my purpose for being alive was somehow connected to this place and the vision behind it.

But it wasn't just Auroville that I loved. It was also India itself, the mingling of devotion and living, spiritual seeking and hustling. I loved being in an environment steeped in thousands of years of sacred consciousness, the land whose longing for the divine produced the mystical streams of the yoga traditions. My own desire for freedom and self-realization were awakened and nurtured.

GurujiMa

The first time I went to meet GurujiMa, I got lost on the way. I arrived late and a little frazzled. Her house was in a quiet neighborhood a few minutes outside of town, a wooded street with sidewalks and shaded lawns, two car garages and neat stacks of cordwood waiting for winter. It was far enough out of town to be off the sewer and water lines, but still had streetlights that lit up the neighborhood at night. The house itself was set on a slight rise, nestled among big hemlocks and pines, with a giant oak tree shading the gravel driveway. It was painted a rich dark chocolate brown, and I entered into a small mudroom where I left my shoes.

Inside, the house was a sea of silence. It was quiet, but more than that it was pervaded by a feeling of silence like outer space, like a silence beyond the reach of sound. In the silence was a stillness full of light, pregnant with energy. The thoughts in my mind were suddenly very loud, garishly obtrusive against the backdrop of emptiness. We walked upstairs to a small room and sat on the floor. The window was cracked and birdsong floated in, somehow without disturbing the resonant silence. Inside the room and outside were two different dimensions. The room had a small altar with a candle and a picture of a lamb sitting on a book in a circle of stars on a red background.

I sat down, and she spoke with a voice that echoed the silence. Her words were clear, but they seemed to come through her from somewhere far away. Her eyes were as deep and full as the ocean. She said she saw me in a prior life as a seeker in India, a sannyasin, "one who has laid everything down", wandering with no possessions, living on pilgrimage, in temples, jungles, and caves, searching for truth. She looked into me, and I remembered the yogi on the slopes of Arunachala. His penetrating gaze joined with hers and led me into the inner chambers of my own heart. I encountered a vast self there, extending beyond birth and death.

After this meeting with her, I couldn't speak. The inner reality that she introduced to me didn't connect to my outer life, to my personality. The gulf was too wide. I couldn't form words. Later that day, driving in the car with Corinne, she asked me to share what had happened, but I couldn't.

I couldn't even apologize. The car window was open, and I felt the breeze on my face. The sun was setting behind a bank of pine trees, throwing golden light heavenward.

Silencing the mind is a major focus of many yoga traditions and teachings. The text commonly called The Yoga Sutras of Patañjali begins by defining yoga as "when the mind stops spinning". And in the Bhagavad Gita, Krishna tells the great warrior Arjuna that a yogi transcends sorrow and pain and finds contentment and the highest happiness by controlling the mind and the activity of the senses. "Like an unflickering lamp in a windless space, the one who has subdued their thoughts practices the yoga of the soul." This kind of mental silence is hard to imagine. When we try to quiet the mind, it resists, evading our grasp. Every thought that we try to quash seems to shatter into ten more thoughts, filling the mind with activity.

On the way to Auroville, the study abroad group I was traveling with stopped for 10 days at Thich Naht Hanh's monastery, Plum Village, in the South of France. I had tried meditating before, sitting still with my eyes closed and listening to the sound of my breath, until suddenly I was off following a train of thoughts, leaping from a childhood memory of feeding a horse a carrot to wondering about why carrots are orange, why nothing rhymes with orange, why it is that rhyming is so pleasing to listen to and so helpful in remembering things, forgetting completely about the horse and the carrot, and then suddenly realizing that I'd wandered far from my breath and making my way back.

I understood the concept basically, but I'd never tried sitting still for any more than 20 minutes at a stretch. At Plum Village, we awoke every morning and went to the meditation hall, where we alternated between sitting, walking, and chanting for at least an hour. This was the first time I'd really come face to face with the intertwined swirls of thoughts that populate my mind.

What is Yoga?

By the second day at Plum Village, I was full of agitation. A few of us went out running through the vineyards of Bordeaux, and I felt like I could run forever. When I sat still, I wanted to squirm out of my skin. My thoughts were endless, obsessive, intrusive. They bloomed, whirled, and divided, streaking like comets across the sky of my consciousness. But over time, I began to discern that there was a sky that the thoughts were moving across. There was a silent, clear backdrop that was holding and containing and witnessing all the chaotic motion. As I got to know my inner sky, my nervous system calmed down and my body was less agitated.

The silence that I experienced in GurujiMa's house had the same quality as this inner sky, but it was outside me. I'd felt this kind of silent stillness before in the inner chamber of the Matrimandir, in the courtyard where Mother and Sri Aurobindo's bodies are buried, and in the aura of a *sādhu* that I'd encountered on the slope of Arunachala. I recognized this feeling. It was like a vibration, a low, subtle hum that pervaded the space and resonated inside me, drawing me to vibrate in sync with it. Just like the Arunachala *sādhu's* own inner stillness provided a clear reflection in which to see what was going on inside me, the silence of her own being radiated out of GurujiMa and filled the house. It made meditation easier, creating a base note that I could harmonize with, a pillar that I could lean on for support as I sought the silence within me.

I could sense that inside, GurujiMa was situated, fixed in that silent stillness. Her mind was not spinning. Like an unflickering lamp, her inner being burned straight upward, radiating warmth and light. She had achieved a state of yoga.

The texts and traditions of yoga describe practices that support movement along a path of yoga that leads to a state of yoga. Different traditions say different things about the path. For some it must be beaten down by a yogi's own will and perseverance, using physical austerities like holding intense postures for long periods of time, extensive fasting, breath retention, and profound mental concentration. The Yoga Sutras say that a yogi achieves yoga through *abhyāsa*, continuous practice over a long period of time, and *vairāgya*, not engaging with emotional attachments or aversions. Over time, austerity practices hone concentration and create space between the mind and the body's cravings and impulses, leaving the inner space clear and quiet. This was the vibe at the Mount Madonna Center. Babaji's patent answer to almost any question about how to progress in yoga was "daily *sādhana*, daily practice".

Other texts and traditions say that a yogi achieves yoga by divine grace. They say that the best practices are those that cultivate the longing to merge with God, those that lead us to call out ever more fervently for love from the Divine Beloved. This longing for God draws lover and Beloved together, and once we catch a hint of that Divine fragrance, all other lesser desires fall away. Once we touch God, thoughts dissolve and we are illuminated by the vast, silent expanse of cosmic consciousness.

Tantrasāra, an incredible text by the great 10th century guru Abhinavagupta that summarizes the core of his tantric teachings, describes the ultimate reality, the foundational essence of existence as the endless radiance of Siva. This pure, infinite light is what we are, what all of creation is, but we don't know that because Siva hides Himself from us. *Tantrasāra* describes the ways that Siva reveals Himself, thus bestowing awakening. The first is *anupāya*, without means. "This person of broad vision enters immediately into self-manifest Siva."

The text then goes on to describe various *upāyas*, or means and methods that Siva provides us for discovering Him by purifying our thoughts so that we can see perfectly clearly. These include various techniques and practices like textual study, *prānayama*, *mantra* recitation, and *nyāsa* practice, through which seed sounds are installed in different places of the body. Tantrasāra accepts both progressive and spontaneous awakening, and weaves them together with the understanding that yoga is achieved through both effort and grace. Each person's path of awakening is unique

What is Yoga?

to them, determined by their unique purpose in this particular lifetime, how far they've progressed in previous incarnations, and how much karmic baggage they're carrying.

GuruijiMa's awakening was *anupāya*. It happened suddenly. She says that it was like being asleep for her entire life, and then suddenly waking up. She had been a wife and mother, a PhD, and vaguely interested in spirituality. But one day the veil fell away and revealed a multidimensional reality that remained stable and consistently visible. She knew that God was real, that life was purposeful, and that there are countless beings of light supporting and nurturing our growth at all times. This knowing didn't fade or flicker. It remained as real as the feeling of sun on your skin.

She was also not part of a yogic lineage. Sometimes yoga teachings were passed down orally from teacher to student in an extended line of what's called the guru-shishya parampara, or teacher-student succession. But not every guru was part of a direct lineage. Throughout India's history, some spiritual luminaries awakened spontaneously, or were even born with access to the state of yoga that others might strive toward for a lifetime.

The famous 7th Century Tamil child-saint Thirugnana Sambandar is said to have composed 16,000 devotional hymns to Siva that touch on the subtlest aspects of bhakti yoga before his death at the age of 16. When he was just three years old, his father went under water during a ritual bath, and he cried out in fear. Lord Siva and his wife Parvati heard his cry and came to console him. When his father surfaced and saw a dribble of milk on his chin, he asked the boy where it came from, and Sambandar sang out a gorgeous song that's now called Todudaya Seviyan. "He wears a ring in his ear and rides on the holy bull...the ash-smeared thief who stole my heart, the One to whom the Creator prays."

Other well-known gurus have experienced a kind of spontaneous awakening. When he was 16 years old, Ramana Maharshi saw a corpse and laid down on the floor to see what death was like. His ego died, and shortly afterward he left home to live in and around Arunachala. Anandamayi Ma performed her own ceremony of spiritual initiation with no prior instruction at the age of 26. She later stated, "As the guru I revealed the mantra; as the disciple. I accepted it and started to recite it." And as a young girl living in a rural fishing village in Kerala, the hugging saint Amma would frequently go into states of ecstatic union with God, much to her family's dismay.

I met GurujiMa roughly 20 years after her initial awakening, and at the time she taught mostly in the Judeo-Christian spiritual tradition. She had never studied yoga or encountered a guru, but I recognized in her the state that I'd read so much about, the state of yoga that is the aim of yoga. She wrote that "the purpose of Creation is and was for God to manifest the totality of Divine consciousness within form, and for form to become one with the Divine, completing a 'circle of creation'." She offered a path to align ourselves with this fundamental purpose of Creation and become one with the Divine. I recognized that this path was the same path as yoga.

And beyond any ideas, she herself was the teaching. She embodied sincerity and integrity, compassion, generosity, and surrender. The radiance of her own divinity poured through the transparent vessel of her human form. She pointed out the path, walked on it herself, and transmitted the energy of her own self-realization. Her body was a vehicle for transformation.

Arunachala

About a month into our time in Auroville, we took a trip to Tiruvannamalai, home of the sacred mountain Arunachala. Arunachala has been a pilgrimage site for millennia, and is understood to be the physical embodiment of Siva, the primordial yogi, the source from which the river of yogic wisdom flows. Looking at Arunachala from the west, you can see what resembles an upturned face with dreadlocks flowing out on either side. And from a certain place on the eastern slope, you can see a rock formation that looks exactly like the foot of a divine dancer, similar to the upraised foot of the ubiquitous Nataraja statue found in yoga studios throughout the world.

Arunachala is beautiful. It rises out of a dusty plain planted with flower and peanut fields, reaching toward the open sky. There's a traditional circumambulation route, a path of about 8 miles that circles the mountain, and that affords views from every angle. Every face is different, displaying steep cliffs, rocky crags, and forested slopes. A verse from the Tamil text Tirumantiram exclaims "Anbe Sivam!", Siva is Love! Arunachala embodies that love and radiates it for miles around.

I walked paths tread by countless feet to caves cut into the hillside, caves that have given shelter to generations of spiritual seekers who joined themselves to the holy mountain in search of truth. Sri Ramana Maharshi was the most famous of these, having been featured in Time magazine and inspiring many devotees and admirers from around the world to embrace his simple yet profound yogic inquiry, "Who am I?" Called Bhagavan, or the Holy One by his devotees, he taught that what we normally experience as self, as me and mine, is an illusion that can be overcome by noticing that I am not my body, my beliefs, my thoughts, my friends, my fears, and on and on. Eventually, by casting off identification with all that we are not, we arrive at the realization of what we actually are, radiant, eternal, and beyond any limiting constructs.

We stayed at his *aśram*, Sri Ramanasramam, which sits at the foot of the mountain path. One day I awoke early and went alone for a walk on the mountain, branching off the main trail and wandering on a more narrow path toward the quiet western side, which was shaded from the rising sun. I passed a family of monkeys who were unfazed by my presence. A mother monkey nursed her baby while another combed her child's hair, picking out bugs and eating them. Birds cried out in joy and a radiant blue sky cradled the world.

As I walked, I muttered the *mantra om namah shivāyah* under my breath. My mind watched the mantra, listening to its rhythm and cadence. My heart opened and received the *mantra*, somehow familiar even though the language was new. Every repetition was energizing. The strange sounds pierced me, winding their way deep into my being, connecting to my soul.

As I walked and muttered, I turned a corner and was startled to see a man sitting on a rock right next to the trail, meditating. His hair was knotted into dreadlocks and tied around his head. He wore a piece of cloth wrapped around his waist and a string of large beads hung from his neck and rested on his bare chest. Ash was smeared on his forehead and arms. I stopped when I saw him, and he opened his eyes, which met mine.

Suddenly, I felt completely naked. It wasn't that I felt physically exposed, as much as seen through. My desire to be liked, and willingness to manipulate or put on a show to gain approval, my fear of failure and inadequacy, my shame and self-loathing, even things that I hadn't known about myself, everything was on display. Confronted by greed, lust, loneliness and despair, I felt ugly and wanted to turn away, but I couldn't. Everything that I'd hidden, even from myself, was there for him to see. And yet he didn't flinch. He smiled, but not in mockery. He smiled in friendship, in love. His eyes said, "Yes, I see you, and it's ok. You are worthy of love." All of this probably took place in the span of 5 seconds, but it felt like an hour. It was agonizing, but also freeing. When I eventually did look away and continued walking, the hair on my arms stood on end, and my eyes pricked with tears.

This yogi was probably part of a continuous lineage of seekers that traces back into prehistory. He had likely renounced social life, stepped out of family ties and social obligations, and participated in the death ritual for his former self. His entire life was dedicated to seeking truth. I saw all of that in his eyes: the ancient trail of aspirants, the depth of commitment, the singleness of purpose. It shone from him visibly, tangibly. His was a different yoga than the yoga I'd seen in Auroville. Rather than seeking to create a spiritual society, he had walked away from society altogether. The poetry of his great leap into the unknown tugged at me. He had found something that I longed for. His austerity had delivered a result. I could see it in his eyes.

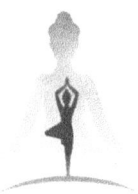

The Evolution of Consciousness and Planetary Transformation

In the modern west, we credit Darwin with "discovering" evolution. But Sri Aurobindo, who lived at a time when Darwin's theories were just beginning to circulate and gain attention, recognized that they were a surface-level articulation of a much deeper cosmic phenomenon. He had studied the *Vedas*, yoga's most ancient texts, and discovered in them hidden teachings that resonated deeply with a comprehensive theory of evolution.

Sri Aurobindo taught that at the base of all manifest reality there is One Single indivisible, eternal, perfect Existence, One Being from which all creation emerges. This One needs nothing, as it is the beginning and end and even the middle of everything that has ever and will ever exist. For the delight of self-discovery, this One has become many, has spun Itself into countless galaxies and solar systems and worlds and beings. All this diversity comes from the One, and actually is made of the One.

And in order to fully immerse in the delight of self-discovery, this One had to completely forget Itself. Eternal consciousness had to become absolute inconscience, all knowledge had to become total ignorance. So the vastness of Eternal Being, called *brahman* in the *Vedas*, the root texts of yoga, cloaked Itself in successive layers of obscurity like a Russian nesting doll. The most superficial, the outermost layer is matter. Inside matter, all the other layers are hidden, and in the center, the deepest layer is the absolute Infinite One, the Divine, God, hiding from Themself in the atoms that comprise the minerals in your bones, in coral reefs, and in the peaks of the Himalayas.

This dive into ignorance was an involution. Then, slowly, over the course of billions of years, a process of evolution peeled away the layers of obscurity. Life, which was hidden within seemingly dead inert matter, emerged. Life invalidated the entropy that governs matter and rejected inertia. It danced in the face of death, organized itself out of chaos. And then the self-aware mind, which had been lying asleep within life, evolved from where it was hiding within life. Mind transcended the individual death of embodied beings, allowing them to live far into the future as stories passed down, words written, accomplishments remembered. Mind doesn't need to eat another mind in order to grow, and it allows for new and radical possibilities of collaboration.

And what else lies within, hiding inside of mind, waiting to evolve? What new capacities will overcome mind's limitations: the linear thought process, the inability to comprehend wholes and the need to objectify something in order to know it? Sri Aurobindo points to a map described in the ancient *Vedas* that shows matter, life, mind, and then an intermediate layer between the lower, limited manifestation and the higher, pure Divine that lies at the heart of all creatures and all creation. This map is reflected in the *Vedas* symbolically as seven rivers (*saptasindhavah* in Rig Veda Samhita) and the seven worlds (*saptalokā* in Taitteriya Aranyaka of Yajurveda).

The higher reality is called *satchitananda*, or being/consciousness/delight. These three aspects describe the qualities of the One that has become

Many. The intermediate layer between the higher and the lower, and the bridge between the two, is called *vijñana*, or gnosis, the wisdom of the heart that knows through identity, that enables an embodied experience of each individual self belonging to the Whole. Sri Aurobindo calls this bridge the supramental consciousness because it is beyond mind, which from our current perspective is the frontier of evolution.

The supramental consciousness is not the mind of steroids. It's not a super or "suped up" version of mind. It's something entirely new, as different from mind as mind is from life. Imagine trying to help a tree understand linguistics or algebra. That's how easy it is for the mental being, whose experience and expectations are defined by thoughts, beliefs, concepts, and linear cause and effect chains, to imagine the supramental consciousness. And yet it is quietly emerging within us as a bridge to self-realization. As we come to experience one human race rather than individual nation states, or as our interdependence on all life begins to replace entitlement to extract resources endlessly from the Earth, we are growing into a supramental awareness. This growth will continue until we see all humans as our family and care for them and the Earth as we would care for a beloved child or sibling.

Evolution traces across billions of years, slowly meandering as nature gradually tries millions of possibilities, hanging on to what works and discarding what doesn't. But evolution traces an exponential curve. The time that it took for mind to evolve out of life is considerably less than the time it took for life to evolve out of matter. And with advances in intercontinental travel and communication, from steam ships to Zoom, we become conscious and intentional participants in our own evolution, and time frames shrink astronomically. Technology grows out of our desire to realize ourselves as one, and it facilitates that realization as well, partly by exposing our inherent interconnectedness, and partly by throwing light on all the times we still act as isolated individuals.

The Divine One secreted Itself within the dense ignorance of matter and then began a process of unveiling through the gradual and intricate processes of Nature. Life emerged from matter, self-regulating and expanding. Then mind emerged from life, with even more capacity for unifying and synthesizing.

And beyond mind is further growth, the evolution of a wisdom that harmonizes opposites, synthesizes truth, experiences the underlying unity of the cosmos. We sit today at the edge of mind's ability to lead us into the future, and a collective call is arising within human hearts for a new capacity that exceeds mind's limitations. This new capacity will change everything: even matter itself will be transformed and divinized as we open to the future. What comes is as radical as the change from plant to fish, or from fish to mammal, or from mammal to human being.

GurujiMa also teaches that we are evolving toward a total realization of our deepest nature. The Divine is living within us as our deepest self, and we are in a gradual process of self-discovery. This process takes place over the course of lifetimes, and is also intertwined with the broader evolution of the Earth itself.

The Earth is not an unconscious rock floating through empty space, but a living evolving being, just like us. She is conscious and her consciousness comprises the consciousness of every being that is part of her. She is awakening, and our individual awakening is totally inseparable from her self-realization.

Evolution is not linear. It surges and recedes, drawing forward in great advances and then settling over long periods of integration and assimilation. GurujiMa teaches that we are currently living through a period of major forward movement, where old patterns of consciousness and behavior are falling away to reveal deeper realizations. The Earth is awakening, passing into a new level of self-understanding, and so is every being that is part of her.

Sri Aurobindo wrote that "There are moments when the Spirit moves among [us] and the breath of the Lord is abroad upon the waters of our being; there are others when it retires and [we] are left to act in the strength or the weakness of [our] own egoism. The first are periods when even a little effort produces great results and changes destiny; the second are spaces of time when much labour goes to the making of a little result."

He called these moments of increased evolution the "Hour of God", which he said "is the hour of the unexpected, the incalculable, the immeasurable." These are times when the evolutionary force is pressing upon on us and compelling transformation. The multiple overlapping and inescapable crises of our time are embodiments of this evolutionary force, drawing us toward something too marvelous to imagine in the current circumstances. The mind cannot fathom what it awaits, feels only the threat of annihilation. But the soul within knows the way through this passage and is sure of the destination.

In the *Rig Veda Samhita*, the root text of the Sanskritic yoga traditions, *Ushā* is the soul of the dawn. She rises each day, casting rays of light into the darkness, transforming the darkness to light. She illumines and awakens. And she is not just an embodiment of the material dawn. She symbolizes the succession of divine dawns that unfold the process of evolution. She "blazes and follows the trail of truth", and she is the "immortal radiant Dawn."

Ushā unveils the new every day, and with every breath. She opens the door to what was impossible yesterday, ushering in the future, taking us over the horizon into uncharted territory. And she is immortal, eternal. She is always arriving, always drawing us forward beyond comfort and familiarity and toward wholeness, harmony and truth. As seekers of truth, we can hitch ourselves to her chariot and allow her to carry us out of darkness and into light.

Yoga is life seeking to expand, to exceed itself. Yoga is the emergent future, the rising sun, the persistent evolutionary movement: from the rock to the plant to the fish, amphibian, reptile, bird, mammal, ape, human… and? Refining and assimilating and attempting, testing an endless variety of possibilities, but always expanding, widening.

Life's emergence from matter was nothing short of miraculous. However it may have happened, a self-organizing, self-individuating, self-preserving tendency developed in the Earth's primordial waters. Bacteria bloomed and joined to create multi-cellular organisms, algae, plankton. Life diversified and expanded, climbing out of the water and fixing itself on land, flowering and flourishing. And as life individuated further, the self-organizing capacity expanded into fish, amphibians, reptiles and mammals, individual untethered beings with proto-brains and proto-egos.

Evolution continued and mind coalesced into a container for consciousness. Mind allows the experience of self as an individual to reach an entirely new level. Mind looks around and sees *not-self* and differentiates that from self. Mind allows the ego, the container of self-identity, to define, refine, and set like a jelly mold. And mind too grows and expands, faster even than life, because now it can grow without killing. Two minds join and build on each other, expanding exponentially. Before writing, the growth of mind was limited by memory and death, but writing extended learning eternally into the future. Before intercontinental travel, mind was limited by perspective and subject to the perimeters of cultural norms, but now the internet has opened the doors to exponential noetic expansion.

Mind has its own limitations. It cannot easily reconcile conflicting ideas; it cannot see wholes, only pieces. It cannot know another being from the inside, only from the outside. And for this reason, it cannot solve any of the critical global social problems that we face today. What can overcome these limitations? What can overstep these bounds?

Every day we take for granted miracles that could not have been fathomed or believed just 200 years ago, not to mention 2,000 or 2,000,000 years. Consider jet planes from a 17th century perspective, or bananas in New England, motion pictures, laparoscopic heart surgery, vaccines, Wikipedia, Google, or video chatting across continents for free. Our consciousness evolves as technologies shrink the world and demolish barriers to experiencing life through the eyes of the "other". We begin to tolerate differences in culture, in life experience, in belief systems, and then protect them, and then celebrate them. The future is emerging, and what is to come will be as unimaginable to our modern sensibilities as mind would have been to a bacterium or a fish or a monkey. Evolution is not over. Evolution is now.

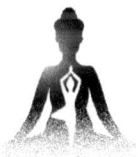

Light and Darkness – Cosmic Forces of Creation

Sri Aurobindo's revelation is profound, nuanced, and multi-faceted. Even he acknowledged that the two major books he wrote about the Vedas (*The Secret of the Veda* and *Hymns to the Mystic Fire*) just begin to scratch the surface and offer a glimpse of their significance. His work has many implications for teaching yoga in the modern west.

He taught that the outer world, the Earth, nature, the ecosystems that contain us, and our inner world are one world, a world that grows increasingly toward wholeness with help from the One Divine being in all Its various manifestations. Many of these various manifestations are embodied as beings that influence our daily life, drawing us along the path of self-realization. This is the same path that the whole Earth travels, as She grows toward the fullest possible realization of Her Divine purpose in the cosmos. The Vedas themselves are hymns to these beings, offering praise and gratitude to them in order to empower them and increase their support for our spiritual growth.

But there are also forces that seek to arrest this growth, forces that seek to increase our sense of separation, isolation, and confusion. The *Vedas* describe a world that is evolving out of darkness and into light, out of ignorance and into knowledge. The advance of light and truth is opposed by forces of darkness and ignorance, but light is stronger and always prevails, not by destroying the darkness by just by being, by growing stronger in its own radiance. The *Vedas* tell us that, in an ancient and Divine collaboration, truth seeks to manifest on Earth and the Earth seeks to manifest truth – the realms of matter and spirit need not be and will not be forever separate.

> "The antinomy between the Light and the Darkness, the Truth and the Falsehood has its roots in an original cosmic antinomy between the illumined Infinite and the darkened finite consciousness. Aditi, the infinite, the undivided, is the mother of the Gods; Diti or Danu, the division, the separative consciousness is the mother of the Titans. Therefore the gods in us move towards light, infinity and unity; the titans dwell in their cave of the darkness and issue from it only to break up, make discordant, wounded and limited our knowledge, will, strength, joy and being."
>
> *The Secret of the Veda by Sri Aurobindo p.421*

Because of the history of white supremacy in religious and moral contexts, it's important to be clear that the force of darkness has nothing to do with skin color. Just like it's hard to see in a dark room, forces of darkness obscure truth. They cast shadows and obfuscate that which would otherwise be clear and visible. Forces of light reveal truth. They illuminate.

Forces of darkness frequently masquerade as light. They pretend to reveal truth, but really they are posing falsehood as truth for the purposes of increasing separation, domination and confusion. White supremacy is an example of this: darkness claims that white skin is superior to darker skin, and claims that this knowledge is a higher truth, only known by some. It equates whiteness with moral and intellectual superiority. In fact, it is entirely untrue and unreal, darkness masquerading as light.

Yoga yokes us to the future. And the future is love. We, in general and as a whole, are becoming more open, more receptive, more caring, more collaborative than humans in the past. Of course, there are forces that push back against this movement. According to Sri Aurobindo's model for understanding, the *Rig Veda*, our universe contains a fundamental tension between forces of light and forces of darkness. Forces of light seek to support and increase truth, while forces of darkness seek to increase falsehood. These forces influence cosmic and global events, as well as the day-to-day events of our individual lives.

> "The Rig Veda rises out of the ancient Dawn with the sound of a thousand-voiced hymn lifted from the soul of [humanity] to an all-creative Truth and an all-illumining Light. Truth and Light are synonymous or equivalent words in the thought of the Vedic seers even as are their opposites, Darkness and Ignorance. The battle of the Vedic Gods and Titans is a perpetual conflict between Day and Night for the possession of the triple world of heaven, mid-air, and earth and for the liberation or bondage of the mind, life, and body of the human being, his mortality or his immortality. It is waged by the Powers of a supreme Truth and Lords of a supreme Light against other dark Powers who struggle to maintain the foundation of this falsehood in which we dwell and the iron walls of these hundred fortified cities of the Ignorance."
>
> *The Secret of the Veda by Sri Aurobindo p.421*

Cosmic Forces in Everyday Life

Yoga is rooted in an ancient spiritual tradition that, in a very nuanced and specific way, describes a world that is much more complex and multidimensional than we typically assume. The *Rig Veda* points to cosmic forces that interpenetrate our individual lives – influencing our thoughts, feelings and beliefs. We are not the isolated beings that we thought we were, enclosed in our skin. Energies, forces of light and darkness, forces that support our growth toward wholeness and forces that seek to block that growth, forces of love and forces of separation move through us, under the radar, but with real effect. Every event in our individual and collective lives can be understood differently through this lens.

Many people today are spiritually starving. We long for connection, for hope, for the experience of being seen and being loved. The *Vedas* tell us that this hunger, this aspiration, is natural. It is not to be ignored or suppressed, but kindled, empowered, and sung out. Our longing for wholeness is as natural as fire, and it purifies us; it burns away separation. It reaches toward heaven and releases an offering of smoke; it lights up the darkness, and it offers warmth and protection. Nurturing our aspiration draws collaborative forces of light to us, empowers them, and transforms life from a chaotic dog-eat-dog scramble to a purposeful adventure of self-discovery.

The multitudinous texts of the yogic traditions are full of interactions between the human, visible world and the world of the invisible: spirits, angels, fairies, demons and ghouls. According to Sri Aurobindo's model for understanding the *Rig Veda*, our universe contains a fundamental tension between forces of light and forces of darkness. Forces of light seek to support and increase truth, while forces of darkness seek to increase falsehood. These forces embody as invisible beings and influence cosmic and global events, as well as the day-to-day events of our individual lives.

Within the context of yoga, the *devas* represent the forces of light. The word *deva* means "shining one", and the devas include Sūrya and Agnī, Indra and Saraswatī, Varuna and Mitra, all of whom are honored in the Rig Veda, as well as Śiva, Vishnu, Brahmā, Durga, Kālī, Parvatī, Ganesh, Murugan, and others whose stories are told in the Mahabharata, the Puranas and other later yogic texts. Each of these unique beings has particular qualities and capacities, and can be invoked to support our yogic quest for truth.

You can find images of the *devas* in songs, statues and stories about them. Someone might give you an amulet for invoking Ganesh, or a mantra, or a picture. All of these external references help us to connect to the being of Ganesh, but none can actually create a relationship of the heart. This requires opening up and calling out, allowing curiosity and a desire to connect to create space for Ganesh in your heart. It requires suspending disbelief and trusting what you feel, see or hear with your inner senses rather than looking for some kind of external sign. Signs may come, but more often the mind translates and twists them into its own language, losing the essence in the process. The heart is more adept at receiving wisdom and love from the devas, which often doesn't come in linear directives but in subtle feelings of rightness, peace and warmth.

Forces of light support our identification and union with our essential self. Light is love and truth absolutely wedded to each other, but it's not an idea; it's a force, a substance, an energy that acts and interacts with our multi-layered selves. Light is embodied in the *devas* of the *Veda*, the beings who seek the highest good for each and for all, and who draw us ever toward the experience of being, giving, and receiving Divine Love. The *devas* nurture experiences of connection, safety, peace, hope and acceptance. They nourish the seeker and empower the search for Truth, reality, wholeness.

Forces of darkness oppose light, and push us toward identification with a separated, isolated ego. Darkness is embodied in the Vedic *asuras, panis* and *dasyus*, who stoke experiences of fear, anxiety, confusion, alienation, loneliness and anger. The *asuras* act on collectives, influencing leaders of national and multinational entities, while the *dasyus* and *panis* act on a smaller scale, but using the same tactics and seeking the same ends. They all work through the ego's vulnerabilities and amplify its sense of separateness. And since we are mostly unconscious of the source of our thoughts, they use thought as a tool to sow confusion and doubt about our divine nature. As we begin to dis-identify with our thoughts, we can watch them move through us, infiltrating from outside, interacting with our own collection of karmic inclinations, and reinforcing the structure of beliefs that forms the ego's fortress and prison.

"Energies of light and darkness exist on cosmic, planetary and individual levels. Light is the primary activating force that moves one toward the further integration of the human and the Divine through a vibrational shift in body and consciousness. Darkness, in its essence, is that which is opposed to the expansion of light. One might wish that only light would be present, guiding the way toward the Divine. However, opposing energies are very common, at times making progress more difficult and creating challenges that need to be overcome. Yet, at the same time, these very challenges enable the self to grow." - *GurujiMa*

The ancient teachings of yoga call to us and invite us to understand ourselves and the world around us more deeply, to pay attention and take notice. The major problems that we face today, personally, locally, nationally, and globally, look insoluble to the separative mechanistic consciousness. But the more we understand the hidden forces that are at play, how they operate and what motivates them, the more possibilities emerge for approaching problems from the inside, by dealing directly with fundamental energies. Then teaching yoga becomes an opportunity to hold a deeper perspective on life and offer it to those who are drawn to you as a guide and friend.

The purpose of human existence, according to Sri Aurobindo, is to collaborate with the devas and forces of light, each an individualized emanation of the Divine One, in the establishment of a "Life Divine" on Earth. This divine life is the culmination of material evolution and the evolution of consciousness (which of course are not separate). And it encompasses all of life, including matter itself, which will progressively become divinized, awakened, and self-luminous. Our collective *dhārma* is to seek out the illumined ones who point the way to greater truth and yoke ourselves to them, allowing them to draw us forward into a fuller and truer version of ourselves.

> "The illumined ones yoke their minds and their thoughts to Him Who is Illumination, Largeness, and Clarity. Knowing all phenomema, He alone orders the energies of the sacrifice. Savitrī, the divine Creator, is vastly affirmed in all things."
>
> Rig Veda V.81.1

Sūrya: The Sun

Sūrya is a leader of the Vedic legions of light. He is the Sun, and just as with *Agni* and the other Vedic devas, *Sūrya* has a physical form that we can see and feel via our external senses, but he is also a Being that encompasses and contains more than the material. We can touch *Sūrya* with our inner senses through the emotions that the Sun evokes in us, through a range of solar symbols and metaphors, and by opening directly to his essence, or soul qualities.

Agni's qualities are heat, light and purification. *Sūrya* shares these qualities, but they are both vaster and more distant, more radiant but less within our control. He is praised in *Rig Veda* Book 1 as "the highest Light of all," and in Book 10 as "all-seeing Intelligence," and "the far-seeing eye of knowledge." He is both illumination, the radiance through which darkness and falsehood are dispelled, and he is the seer that perceives the truth, discerning the real from the unreal, knowledge from ignorance. Sri Aurobindo calls *Sūrya* "the light of the Truth rising on the human consciousness." *Sūrya* "goes where the gods have made a path for him." The other devas support us, releasing the hold that ignorance has placed upon us. *Sūrya*, following in their wake, pours down from above the infinite light of truth.

> "Sūrya, the Sun, is the master of [the] supreme Truth–truth of being, truth of knowledge, truth of process and act and movement and functioning. He is therefore the creator or rather the manifester of all things, for creation is outbringing, expression by the Truth and Will, and the father, fosterer, enlightener of our souls. The illuminations we seek are the herds of this Sun who comes to us in the track of the divine Dawn and release and reveal in us night-hidden world after world up to the highest Beatitude."
>
> *Hymns to the Mystic Fire by Sri Aurobindo p,31*

Sūrya is also known by other names which are applied to his specific qualities. *Savitrī* is the Creator, the Awakener, the divine action of light that penetrates darkness and opens new possibilities. *Savitrī* illumines our consciousness, stirs aspiration within us, awakens us from the dream that we had mistaken for reality. *Savitrī* plants the seeds of tomorrow in today's soil, and then coaxes them out of their husks, drawing their tendrils up through the crust of earth and into the open air.

om bhur bhuvah svah
tat savitur vareniyam bhargo devasya dhimahi
diyo yo nah pracodayāt.

> "Om, Earth, Heaven, and the Region Between. We fix our consciousness on the glorious Savitrī, purifying radiance of the devas. Please illuminate our minds."
>
> *-The Gayatri Mantra: Rig Veda Mandala III, Sukta 62, Mantra 10*

Pūshan is another aspect of *Sūrya*. He is the Increaser, day-by-day fostering, nourishing, expanding our consciousness and capacity to embody truth. *Pūshan* embodies the evolutionary impulse, reaching ever higher, climbing through the ages and always increasing, expanding, widening. He is the force of purification that clears away the darkness that clings to us, flushing it out from hiding and into the light of day. *Pūshan* is our experience of Truth that grows with each new dawn and never recedes, expands ever toward the horizon, encompasses more and more of the infinite sacred wholeness that underlies everything everywhere. *Sūrya* does not just disappear into the depth of night and reappear each morning in an endless static cycle. Each dawn is new, entirely unlike any dawn that has come before, breaking ground and ushering in the future.

This tension between light and darkness exists in the universe, and it also influences both the macrocosm of geopolitical events and the microcosm of our individual lives. If we seek to understand ourselves, to discover our essential nature and embody truth in our daily lives, then we will gain a great deal from understanding the hidden forces that inform our desires, our aversions, our aspirations, and our fears. For what we typically think of as our *self* is actually an agglomeration of forces and voices, each with its own agendas and aims, jostling and wrestling with each other in an effort to control our thoughts and actions. The ego itself is a veil that hides the individuality of these forces behind a gathered sense of *I, me, mine*. And as long as the essential self (*purusha*, soul, spirit, *jīvātman*, etc.) remains hidden and subdued, our lives are a battlefield for these forces.

> "A superconscient Truth lies concealed and is the basis of the infinite being which stands revealed on those higher altitudes of our ascension…[W]e have to bring forward the Truth as an offering so that the luminous god with his golden hands full of the Light may rise high in our heavens and hear our word…[W]e must widen out the cord of Savitrī so that it shall release us into higher states of life made accessible to us and harmonized within our being."
>
> *The Secret of the Veda by Sri Aurobindo p.437*

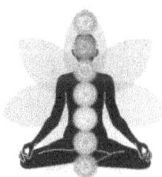

Yajña - The Vedic Sacrifice

We have covered the first two foundational elements of the cosmology of yoga that is the basis for this book. First, we are living in an evolving universe. The Divine One has become many and limited Its eternal being, consciousness, power, knowledge and delight. The One plunged into the depths of matter, and the evolution of consciousness is Its process of remembering.

Second, this cosmos contains beings and forces that support and nurture this process of evolution, and beings and forces that inhibit it. These beings and forces interact with the Earth and humanity, though we are mostly unaware of their influence. They influence our thoughts and ideas, our feelings and emotions, and our state of physical health and vitality.

Matter emerged from the empty void, and life evolved out of matter. As life emerged, it organically sought to expand, diversify, and reflect the infinite nature of its source in the One. But life could not expand infinitely. Death sought to snuff it out, and the force of death is always chasing life.

Single celled bacteria diversified and transformed, and eventually life took more complex forms. The seas gave birth to fungi, jellyfish, whales, frogs, turtles, iguanas, birds, mice, cats, elephants, and monkeys. Along the way, mind grew slowly in the background, shaping itself and preparing for its more full emergence in humans. As mind emerged from within life, it naturally sought Truth, the infinite, perfect, absolute Truth. But mind cannot discover perfect Truth. It cannot penetrate the surface, so it breaks Truth into fragments and tries to understand the pieces. It confuses the part with the whole, and brokenness with unity.

In the presence of falsehood and death, a special protective power arose within humans. This power creates the experience of being individual, of being enclosed in a container that defines what is me and what is not me. In the yoga tradition, this power was called *ahankara*, "that which creates I-ness". *Ahankara* serves the purpose of creating a sense of safety in an unpredictable world, and of creating a sense of continuity for a self that is constantly changing.

As the destination of the yogic path, the true self is written about extensively in the texts of the yoga tradition. Its nature is explored and described, as well as the difference between the true self and the false self, the persona that most of us identify as 'I' and 'me'. In a compressed (*laghu*) version of the Yoga Vāsishtha (4.3), a text that contains a conversation between the divine human Rāma and his *guru* Vāsishtha, Rāma asks Vāsishtha about the nature of *ahankāra*, the 'I-maker'.

Vāsishtha replies that there are three levels of *ahankāra*. The first level knows that all the world and the Supreme Soul is my eternal self. The second level realizes that who/what I actually am is more subtle than the tip of a germ of rice, ever-existent, and beyond creation. He notes that these two *ahankāras* are always beneficial, but the third *ahankāra* is terrible and should be destroyed at all costs. This third *ahankāra* identifies myself with my body and brain alone.

As long as I believe and experience myself to be only this body and the thoughts produced by this brain, I am wholly controlled by need and greed, fear and clinging. I am, as Vāśishtha says, seized by the unreal idea of 'me' and 'mine'. The needs of the body are my needs, and they must be satisfied over the needs of any other bodies. I am in competition for survival, and domination is the only solution. I must protect myself, manipulate, steal, and hoard. This may sound extreme, but if you look at the people who our society rewards with admiration and control of resources, it tends to be those who dominate others and hoard wealth.

Ahankāra is often translated as 'ego' because it is what creates our individual sense of identity, or experience of being a self that is different, separate from our environment, and unique. But we have to remember that when the ancient yogis were discussing and exploring the nature of *ahankār*, Freud was thousands of years away. Our current understanding of the word ego is overlaid with lots of concepts from modern psychology that would not have been intended or understood in the word *ahankāra*. We tend to think of ego as something selfish, greedy, lustful and petty. We hear about building a healthy ego or taming the ego as if it's a circus animal or a pet. But the sense of the word *ahankāra* is simpler. It's essentially like a magnet that draws the vast, cosmic self-awareness into a point of individuality. It's the container that holds the experience of 'I' as distinct from 'you' or 'that'. According to the yoga traditions, consciousness is like a vast, unified sea, and *ahankāra* just makes it seem individuated.

This experience of individuation is raw and vulnerable. As an individual, I feel cut off from the ecosystem around me, competing for survival against a cold and heartless world. Experiences of love soften the edges of isolation, but they only go so far. As long as I'm identified with this bounded body and brain, I need to find a way to navigate this world and get my needs met.

The eternal, omnipotent, omniscient One has diversified Itself into countless souls, and these souls have consented to be encapsulated in individuality, wrapped up in an experience of isolation. These souls have agreed to be immersed in the delusion of separateness, separated from the purpose for their existence, forgetful of their true nature, and subject to physical pain and limitation. The ego has replaced the soul as the axis of identity in the ecosystem of delusion, and it is programmed with a need for self-preservation.

We naturally want to survive, and we want to maintain the stability of our sense of self. But realizing who we actually are requires that we transcend identification with the ego. We have to let go of our seemingly stable, reliable sense of self in order to experience a much more stable, eternal, radiant self that can never be harmed or killed. In order to find the truth, we have to sacrifice the delusion that has helped us cope with life as it is.

And so we come to the third element of our cosmology of yoga. The conception of *yajña*, or sacrifice, is central to the *Vedas*. The outer form of the ritual called *yajña* or *homa* involves a Vedic priest building a fire according to very specific parameters and then chanting specific mantras while making offerings to the fire. Everything is prescribed, and often the ritual is done with a specific purpose in mind. Some *mantras* and offerings are intended to generate wealth, or health, or success in school or business.

But the inner meaning of the *yajña* is not about material gain. The inner meaning is about relationship. When we make an offering, we are acknowledging relationship. The *yajña* honors the four directions, the five elements, the body of the Earth and the celestial beings that love us and support our evolution. It invokes them and invites them to participate in our life more directly. It asks them to bless us not with material riches but with self-knowledge, humility, and the delight of belonging to all that exists.

In order for any whole to function properly, its constituent parts have to sacrifice their individuality. The parts have to work together and value the working of the whole over their separate benefits. This is as true in our bodies as it is in government, in sports teams, or in schools of fish. The individual has to place the good of all over its own needs. The delusion that my needs are more important than our needs can only persist for so long. Eventually the system breaks down and we all suffer.

The *Rig Veda Samhita*, root text of the Sanskritic yoga traditions, begins with a hymn to *agni*, the being of fire:

agnimīle purohitam yajñasya devāmritvijam hotāram ratnadhātaram

> "I adore Agni, the flame, priest of the sacrifice, the shining and righteous one who calls forth infinite spiritual wealth."
>
> *- Rig Veda 1.1.1*

In the ritual yajña performed by vedic priests, fire is central. Offerings are made to the fire and mantras are sung to the fire. Participants in the ritual circle the fire and bow to the fire. This outer fire represents the inner flame of aspiration that burns in every heart, the flame that empowers the evolution of forms and consciousness. The first hymn of the *Rig Veda* praises this fire, the soul of fire itself, that accepts our offerings of confusion, fear, doubt and frustration. The flame of aspiration, the desire to know ourselves and the divine, which lives within our deepest heart accepts and transforms all of our limitations, purifying and releasing them upward toward the heavens. The heavens receive the smoke of our burnt offerings and release the gift of grace, raining down blessings upon us.

Agni is the priest of our personal sacrifice, the mediator between us and God. He blazes always upward and devours all that is temporary, leaving behind the essence, the ash, the *vibhuti*. He is warm and comforting and also too hot to touch, inhabiting the space between human and divine, burning all that maintains that division. He sings a holy song, calling out to the beings of light that guide our growth toward wholeness.

In book 10 of the *Rig Veda*, the *Purusha Suktam* describes the primordial creator, "that splendid being born before the beginning of time" as being offered into the sacrificial fire. It describes how all things were created from this sacrifice, the Soul of All offering Itself to the fire so that the world as we know it could come into being.

In the *Bhagavad Gītā*, Krishna tells Arjuna that "with sacrifice the primordial creator created all beings and said, 'By this shall you also create'." Within the yoga traditions, sacrifice is commonly understood to be central to the continuance of life on Earth. Each new birth is a sacrifice, each death is a sacrifice, and with every breath we exhale an offering and inhale a blessing.

The word sacrifice has made its way into our modern lexicon with the insinuation of letting go of something that we care about, giving something up. But truly sacrifice is not a loss, it is a gain. By releasing the ego's perceived needs, beliefs, preferences and fears, we open ourselves to a greater experience of who we actually are. We are used to thinking of ourselves in terms of what we enjoy, what we believe, what we avoid, and what we need in order to feel safe and secure. Letting them go means stepping into the unknown and asking, who am I actually? This sacrifice is the root of yoga.

For the soul, which is inherently free, eternal and unified with all that is, embodiment as a human in the realm of duality is inherently a sacrifice. We forsake the infinite freedom, knowledge, immortality, and bliss of our souls and incarnate into limitation, ignorance, death, and suffering in the process, forgetting our true nature. What could be worse? Why would we choose such a thing? From the standpoint of the ego, it's impossible to imagine why one would give up eternal delight for a life of confusion and swinging between happiness and sadness, enjoyment and pain.

But the soul understands the true nature of sacrifice, and that the whole universe was created through sacrifice, is sustained through sacrifice, and grows and changes through sacrifice. Escape from sacrifice is impossible, and seeking escape only leads to deeper suffering. Each soul has willingly chosen self-giving in order to participate in the delight of becoming, the joy of self-discovery.

When we shift from a self-identity as the limited and self-isolated ego to a self-identity as an immortal soul, we gain a wider perspective on the sacrifice itself. The soul gives itself willingly to life, consenting to participate in the collective evolutionary endeavor of the Earth's awakening. The Earth offers itself without reserve to every soul, and every soul offers itself to the Earth. The individual good that a separated consciousness holds so dear is released in favor of the collective good that embraces not just all of humanity, but all of life and beyond. We are not the victim of the sacrifice, but the Lord of the sacrifice, willingly offering all that we are in service of the Oneness that is God.

> "'Sacrifice' and 'letting go' of something one values are often considered to be the same thing. However 'letting go' can take place along many lines of motivation and for many purposes, whereas the deepest meaning of 'sacrifice' is to 'make sacred', a choice that involves the soul. To 'sacrifice' something is to let go of something or to endure or bear the pain of something in order to further the purposes of a higher ideal that partakes of the Divine. It is in service to this higher ideal that one gives up something precious in order to bring something even more precious into being."
> — ***GurujiMa***, <u>Sacrifice and the Soul's Choice</u>

A Divine Life on Earth means the freeing of matter, life and mind from their inherent limitations. It means that matter will no longer decay, life will no longer feed upon itself, and mind will open to a direct perception of unity. This evolutionary process has been going on and will continue whether you or I consciously participate with it or not. But the next evolutionary phase includes the collective awakening of humankind to our hidden *dhārma*, the holy task lying quietly within our deepest hearts, and a joining in collaboration with the forces of Light to establish love and truth on the Earth.

When we harness ancient sunlight to power our modern conveniences, or derive vaccines and medicines from plants and micro-organisms, mind is shaping life and matter. Similarly, life and mind will be transformed by the influx of new potential that comes through this collaboration with the forces of Light. The transformation of matter is taking place right now, in the energetic substructure of dirt, rocks, water and plants, and of course within our own bodies. This is something we can sense, feel, experience if we can release old habits of thinking and pay attention to our bodies with clear, innocent attention. Every breath offers us a doorway to direct experience of our body's cells and systems waking up to their own divinity.

Yoga is union, joining the individual with the collective, the collective with the whole, and the whole with the infinite from which it arises. The *Rig Veda* provides the context for understanding many subsequent yogic texts. Its symbology is used as a foundation and is expanded upon throughout the *Upanishads*, *Purānas*, *Rāmāyana*, *Mahābhārata*, and others. If we apply Sri Aurobindo's interpretation of the Veda to the dramas of these later compositions, they become practical guidebooks for navigating a purposeful life in a multidimensional universe. They support the journey of yoga.

> "When your [emotional] being consents to give up its desires and enjoyments, when it offers itself to the Divine, then the Yajna will have begun... It doesn't mean that you give up all works for the sake of the Divine – for there would be no sacrifice of works at all. Similarly the sacrifice of knowledge doesn't mean that you painfully and resolutely make yourself a fool for the sake of the Lord. Sacrifice means an inner offering to the Divine and the real spiritual sacrifice is a very joyful thing."
>
> – *Sri Aurobindo*, <u>Letters on Yoga, Book One</u>

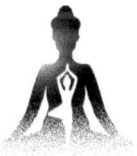

The Process of Purification

There is a narrative going around in the modern yoga world that says that purification is bad, and that yoga doesn't involve purification. This narrative says that we are fine the way we are, and we don't need to change. This is a new idea, and does not resonate with actual teachings of yoga from historical texts and traditions.

What this narrative is really pointing to is the fact that many of us in the modern world use self hatred as a vehicle for change. We judge ourselves and find ourselves lacking, and use this dissatisfaction as momentum to work out or study so we can be stronger and smarter and more beautiful. But self hatred is not the only motivator. We can desire to be more loving, more truthful, more sincere, and more humble. We can be changed by love, hope, and aspiration. These changes are purification, and they happen naturally to anyone who commits to the path of yoga, if by yoga we mean a realization of the inherent unity of all.

Purification is also misunderstood or misrepresented in modern western yoga because yoga today is frequently used to bolster the ego's false power. It's lumped in with fad diets and cosmetic surgery as a way to make us better, more lovable, worthier. We see what the ego does with the idea of purity and perfection, twisting it to strengthen the walls of its fortress. But true purification, like yoga, is not a means of strengthening the separated, isolated, lonely self. It's not a tool for self-improvement, but a process of profound self-love.

Purification is an essential aspect of yoga. The Hathapradīpika (2.5) defines purification on a physical level, saying that in order to develop the ability to retain *prāna*, all the *nadīs* and *cakras*, which are *malākulam*, or full of impurities, should be śuddhim, or purified. Chapter 2, verse 19, says that when the *nadīs* are purified, the body becomes thin and radiantly beautiful. 2.22 recommends six actions which include swallowing a strip of cloth and pulling it back up to clear out the stomach and esophagus, enemas to clear the intestines, flossing a thread between nose and mouth, unblinking gazing, abdominal massage, and bellows breath. All of these actions have the effect of cleansing the physical body of impurities, or that which would inhibit the body's natural processes of homeostasis.

Of course, since modern yoga has merged with the fitness industry, it's easy for these teachings to be taken out of context and appropriated by the ego. We are deluged with messages about how we should look, and we learn young that how we look determines opportunities and access to resources. We are inclined to want to be thin and radiantly beautiful. The danger is that these teachings were not developed for the ego's benefit. They were developed to support conditions for transcending the ego and experiencing the deeper Self that lies beyond ego. What we put into our bodies affects our consciousness and our ability to see clearly. So physical purification, while not the only consideration in yoga, is at least a valuable one.

The great tantric teacher Abhinavagupta also wrote about purification. In the first chapter of Tantrasāra, or "the essence of tantra", he wrote, "The śāstras (sacred texts) describe *ajñāna* (ignorance) as the cause of bondage.

Ajñāna is known as *mala* (impurity). Perfect knowledge completely uproots *mala*. When all *malas* are destroyed, one attains *moksha* (liberation)."

Abhinavagupta's focus is not on impurities in the body, but impurities in the mind. Tantrasāra describes several ways to purify the *vikalpas* (thought constructs) that lead us to believe that we are bound and not free. These ways include hearing the truth from a guru, meditative concentration, working with *prāna*, and specific practices with *mantra* and *nyāsa*.

True reality is unlimited, undivided consciousness, a total oneness of all that exists in form and all that is formless. Our thought constructs include not just thoughts themselves but beliefs, mental models, perspectives, ideas. They are the lenses through which we view ourselves and the world. And they create the experience of limitation and division. When they are purified, we realize that we are free and one. This is the essence of tantra, according to Abhinavagupta.

Again, the ego can easily appropriate these teachings and make them about aggrandizement. We can think about what we'll get if we purify our minds, how we'll be free and powerful and able to accomplish all our goals and defeat our enemies. But the fundamental innate radiance of being that Abhnavagupta tells us is our true nature is not ego. Ego doesn't win anything through yogic purification. In fact it loses the illusion of personal power and control. These illusions are sublimated into the true reality, which is that all power belongs to the One, and only through union (*yoga*) with that One can we have any power at all. The power that is then achieved is not power over anything, but the power of being everything.

Krishna in the Bhagavad Gita also teaches Arjuna that yoga is a path of purification. In the fifth chapter, he says that the yogi who is *yogayukto* (yoked to yoga) and *viśuddhātma* (whose self is purified), whose self has become the Self of all things, remains pure even when acting. By giving up the fruits of their actions and realizing that they are not the "doer" of

The Process of Purification

their actions, yogis enter a process of *atmaśuddhaya* (self-purification). Here we have a direct articulation that the ego's claim on the results of what we do is a primary obstacle to *yoga*.

In the Mundaka Upanishad, the guru Angiras tells his student Śaunaka that the indivisible Self, which is the Supreme treasure, the bright and pure Self, the birthless One without a second, reveals Itself after the mind has been *viśuddha*, purified. And even when they don't use the specific word, purification is a central theme of all the primary Upanishads. They teach that what truly we are, beneath the experience of limitation and duality, is eternal radiant Oneness, united with all that has form and all that is formless. When we release all the obscurities that inhibit our vision, we realize that truth and become it.

Patañjali, in the Yoga Sutras, also teaches a path of purification. He advocates *citta prasādanam*, or purification of consciousness as a way of achieving equanimity (1.33). And he says that when we are able to unify our consciousness, our memory is purified and our true nature shines forth unobstructed (1.43). He offers śauca, or purification, as one of the five *niyamas*, or personal disciplines that are central to yoga. Śauca is also included in Narada's Bhakti Sutras as an integral part of the path of *bhakti*, or devotional love.

As with many yogic teachings, the word śauca can be used and understood on many levels. It can refer to the physical purification methods taught in the Hathapradīpikā and other Hatha Yoga texts like the Gherandasamhitā. And it can refer to keeping one's physical space clear. Śauca can also imply keeping one's thoughts and intentions clear and sincere, and not getting involved with messy emotional dramas. It essentially points to the purity of our being and encourages us to seek that purity, live in it, align with it, and attend to all the habits that pull us out of it and into illusion.

Looking back at yoga's history, we see traditions of self-mortification and self-denial that flowed from Shankara's doctrine of *māyā-vāda*. *Māyā-*

vāda holds that all form is illusion, and that we should endeavor to escape the illusion by rejecting our bodies, our material lives, and our family/social ties to identify totally with the pure immortal oneness. Yogis in the *māyā-vāda* tradition leave society and practice self-deprivation and self-mortification (literally killing the self) as an approach to purification.

But the Divine One created this form and is this form. From the *Isha Upansihad*, "All this that moves within the moving universe is for the Lord's habitation." And the *Taittirriya Upanishad*, "Itself created itself; none other created it. And so it is called beautiful. And this that is beautifully made, it is no other than the Delight behind existence." If we reject the form of our bodies or the form of our lives as essentially illusory, then we reject that One Who is that form.

At the same time, we do find that we are immersed in delusion. We are surrounded by confusion about what's real, what's true, what's good and wholesome. We live in an evolutionary universe where the Divine One is emerging from the depths of ignorance and separation toward the expanse of truth and unity. We are this evolution; our collective awakening is the re-union of the One Divine Beloved with itself in the form of many Divine Beloveds.

Purification is a central aspect of the path of yoga, and has been considered as such by teachers from many different lineages. The centrality of purification is mentioned in texts from the hatha yoga, tantrik, vedanta, raja yoga, and bhakti yoga traditions. It appears in the Puranas and the Itihasa, as well as the śruti texts. This is because yoga is essentially a path of self-realization, and the first step on the path is to acknowledge that we are headed somewhere that we have not yet arrived. We are moving in a direction, toward a destination.

Yoga is a path, a process, a journey, as well as a state of being. The state of yoga is the state of complete realization of who we are. It is the state in which our consciousness unifies with the essential consciousness that

The Process of Purification

permeates all, and in which we see no "other" outside of ourselves, only different manifestations of the oneness that we are. This is a basic state of love that cannot be broken or harmed. When I am all, I cannot but love all, and as long as the state persists the love cannot diminish.\

As long as I'm on the path of yoga, headed toward the state of yoga, there will be obstacles that prevent me from knowing who I am and experiencing the unity of all. These obstacles block me from knowing my pure being. They are impurities that need to be removed in order to reveal the purity.

If my ego takes up the mantle of purification for its own ends, then I will try to create and control the process, and I will measure my progress based on selfish standards. Am I beautiful enough? Am I strong enough? Am I smart or fearless or flexible enough? I will judge myself and perhaps hate myself for not measuring up. But this self hatred is itself an impurity.

The purity of my deeper being does not win. It does not dominate or control. It just shines like the sun. Shadows may encroach, but it does not fight. It just continues shining, and its brilliance progressively dissolves that which obscures its shining. We don't achieve purity, we surrender to it. We release all that stands in its way. We offer our impurities to it and allow them to be transformed. This is the path and process of yoga.

The *Pavamāna Abhyāroha* is a beautiful prayer that appears in the *Brihadaranyaka Upanishad* (1.3.28):

asato mā sad gamaya,
tamaso mā jyotir gamaya,
mṛtyor mā amṛtaṃ gamaya

Pavamāna is a word that appears throughout the *Rig Veda* in the context of purification. And *abhyāroha* has a sense of an ascending prayer of devotion. This prayer of purification is a calling out to be led (*gamaya*) from falsehood (*asat*) to truth (*sat*), from darkness (*tamas*) to light (*jyoti*), from death (*mrityu*) to immortality (*amrita*).

Purification is the falling away of the impurity of ignorance that clouds our vision. As we release identification with thoughts, ideas, preferences, habits, relationships, and other self-definitions, we are left with the essential truth of being that breathes us into existence. This essential truth is not emptiness. It is not negative, but absolutely positive and full. It is the pure delight of being, the joy of existing, dancing our unique dance, singing our unique song.

Spiritual purification is not self-destructive. It is loving and nurturing. If you find a child covered in blankets, suffocating beneath the weight, the most loving act is to begin taking off the layers that keep the child trapped. So it is with your essential self, or ātman. Ātman is the deepest and truest you, the one that is covered in blankets and aching to breath and be free. And purification is the process of peeling away the layers of falsehood that obscure your natural radiance.

This requires discernment, but we need not face it alone. Prayer acknowledges that purification is a partnership between ātman and *brahman*, between the individual and God. Without this partnership, we are left with the ego in charge. To paraphrase Ramana Mahārshi, the great 20th century sage of Arunachala, when the thief is made the policeman, there will be plenty of investigation, but no arrests. Even as we experience ourselves as a limited individual self, enclosed within the walls of our own mind, we can call upon and receive support from the vast intelligent Love that holds all within its infinite heart.

Patañjali's Yoga Sutras explain that we come into life carrying some luggage from past lives. We are not clean slates, ready to absorb and mirror our intellectual and emotional environments. We are in the midst of an ongoing journey, and we're carrying energies, impressions, seeds that we've picked up along the way. These seeds lie dormant within our

The Process of Purification

consciousness, waiting for the right environmental conditions to sprout and unfurl the concentrated experience that they carry like a tiny blueprint within them.

Purification is a process that clears out anything that limits our vision, preventing us from seeing the truth of who we are and the truth of God. It doesn't make us bigger, better, smarter, prettier, cleaner, or superior to anyone else. It doesn't feed the ego and its desire for adulation and self-aggrandizement. It squeezes the ego like a wet sponge, wringing out the false sense of importance, the false experience of need for control.

And it's not a linear process. It's not like the car wash, where we go through and come out sparkling. Purification is an iterative, evolutionary journey that takes us deeper and deeper into the unconscious patterns of thinking and acting that keep us trapped in a small, fearful version of ourselves. It dredges up ancient soul trauma and pain that we have buried and carried through lifetimes. Purification is activated by current life circumstances. It happens now, and this is its healing power. It brings the past into the present so it can be faced and released.

Purification is a natural process tied to the evolution of consciousness that underlies all of life. It has its own gravity and momentum. We each carry within us energies that are not light and truth, energies that obscure or hide who we are or seek to prevent our self-realization. These energies are often held in our body tissues and in the field of energy that surrounds us. They influence our fundamental beliefs about reality, our basic ideas about what is safe and what is dangerous, and our preferences and attractions.

The process of purification is activated by spiritual light, the Divine light of creation that empowers evolution. This light is often concentrated in spiritual places, called *tirthas*, or bridges in the yogic traditions. A *tirtha* could be a temple or a mountain, a shrine or a tree, any place that holds spiritual light. Throughout India, millions of *tirthas* are revered as sacred places for ceremonies and prayers, and some are major places of pilgrimage. People will walk for days or months to touch the light in these places.

Spiritual teachers and their writings or recorded words can also carry spiritual light. For one who is seeking, the teachings are like a balm or a nourishing drink. And just being in the presence of a teacher who carries great light can be transformative. This is because the light itself joins with our own inner aspiration to initiate the purification process, drawing latent energies up into our field of awareness and out. When we experience these energies and release them without reacting or acting them out, they are gone from our field and we are more free to embody and express the truth of our deeper being.

Each one of us is clutching a tangle of mental ideas about what's real and possible as well as embodied trauma held in the tissues of our bodies. These ideas and embedded inhibitions combine to shape our personality, our expectations, and our lives. The Divine Beloved is constantly tugging at the tangle, trying to help us get free. Often that tugging manifests as life circumstances that trigger the outpicturing of what we have buried and carried, the karmic root ball that feeds our sense of self. Spiritual light is like an activator that spurs the untangling and opens the way for transformation. But we have to be willing to face the energies that are released and let them go.

When energies of fear that I carry in my bioenergetic field are activated and drawn up into my awareness, I will experience that fear. If I run and hide, get drunk or high, go shopping, or otherwise distract myself from the fear, it will settle back down and await another time to release. But if I can bear the experience and face the fear, allow it to course through me and not avoid it, then it will clear out. The same is true of anger, jealousy, despair, or hatred. An episode of concentrated purification can be short lived and mild or very intense, depending on the intensity and amount of the energy being released. But it always passes.

The Process of Purification

In his extensive summary of yogic wisdom called *Tantrāloka*, the 10th century yogi Abhinavagupta teaches that our limitless and pure essential being, which is Śiva, has freely taken on impurity, which is the root of our suffering. He offers *tantrik* practices as a means of purification, of clearing that which obscures our vision. This purification is not a task taken on by the ego in order to become cleaner, or to become more worthy of love. It is a submission of the ego to a process that strips its reinforced self-delusion and opens the way to an experience of the actual purity that is the Self's true nature.

Thoughts that support the experience of separation and isolation are purified, and since these thoughts are understood to be deeply rooted in the body, the purification process includes physical purification. For purification to truly occur, the aspirant must surrender the personal will to a higher power, since the ego is constructed to resist, and cannot really offer itself to be cleansed of falsehood. It will use powerful manipulations to remain concealed.

> "The very nature of consciousness is its freedom from thought constructs (vikalpa)…Listening to this nature of the Self repeatedly, thinking of it, and meditating on it continuously help the vikalpa to be become purified…With the purification of vikalpas, in the right manner, consciousness shines forth with all its glory."
> – *H.N. Chakravarty's footnote to Chapter 4 of his Tantrasāra translation*

Purification can happen on the level of the mind, the life, and the body. Purifying your mind does not require rejecting your mind; it requires discerning and releasing those thoughts, beliefs, and ideas that are limiting, anti-love, and anti-life, including those that we have inherited through karma, family, or trauma, and those that we take in through movies, books, "news" outlets, etc. Purifying your life does not require leaving behind your work, your family, your friends, and your home; it requires releasing those aspects of work, those relationships, and those attachments that are limiting, anti-love, and anti-life. Purifying your body not require rejecting it, denying its basic needs for food, water, movement, and breath; it requires releasing addiction and attachment to foods and drinks and habits that harm your body and create confusion in your mind and emotions. It requires spending time listening to your body and its innate desire to move and breathe and laugh and cry.

Your body in particular is a field of great promise and great challenge. In modern western culture it is common to live in a dis-embodied way, to live primarily in our minds. Bringing awareness into your body is itself inherently an act of purification, especially when accompanied by prayer. The light of your awareness, joined with Divine Light, begins to penetrate the layers of obscurity held in your body, layers that are not just your own, but are part of the primal obscurity of matter. Entering your body and touching these layers can be uncomfortable. But staying with it, keeping the light of awareness in the body, exploring the layers of physicality and their innate wisdom and beauty, inherently clarifies and purifies your body and illuminates ways of loving and tending to its needs. Unwholesome desires (those that lead away from an experience of wholeness) become more obvious, and we can start to let them go. Unloving behaviors stand out.

We can bring the light of our awareness into our bodies while we move. We can savor the experience of tending to the body, feeling the flow of life force seeping and rushing, pulsing and swirling to nourish and enliven our tissues, organs, glands, bones. Every aspect of the human body is holy, and it seeks to express its vibrancy. The body longs to radiate and join with the ātman in a pure expression of divinity. We can nurture this longing and draw body and ātman into proximity, into relationship, and into yoga (union).

As we go within and explore our inner dimension, we begin to see that thought is not the final frontier. In fact, thoughts can be like clouds in the sky, blocking the sun's radiance. When we pay excessive attention to our thoughts, and allow them to solidify into rigid beliefs, we can develop a

The Process of Purification

thick and unyielding personality that rejects vulnerability. And when we define ourselves based on others' judgments, this dense layer is reinforced and strengthened.

In order to see what's really there we need to soften, become vulnerable, and release the thoughts and beliefs that make up this coating. When we learn to yield our weight to the earth as we move around in our bodies, instead of propping ourselves up using our muscular strength, we gain resilience, relaxed stamina, and comfort. In the same way, when we learn to yield to the Divine One that encompasses and infuses us, letting our sense of self arise from this field of love rather than our habits and conditioning, we gain inner stability, integrity, and grace.

Each life is woven together into a vast fabric where every thought, prayer, word, and action impacts the whole, and thus holds deep meaning. We are entirely integrated into the cosmos, so every movement of heart, mind or body that we make changes everything, including the movement to know ourselves. When we value our inner life, we encourage others to do the same, and support a collective movement toward greater authenticity. This takes commitment in a world that draws us out, encourages us to determine our self-worth based on the judgments of others, and see ourselves from the outside.

But we are meant to live from the inside out – not from the outside in. We are meant to live in the spontaneous and constant flow of truth that pours from the eternal and unchanging One into this world of change. As the truth that is love floods the world of form, all that resists truth is swept away by its irresistible current. This is the vast sweep of evolution, from the big bang to this moment and beyond into the miracle of tomorrow. It's where we are all headed together.

As a yoga teacher, students will come to you looking for both physical practice and practical philosophy, how to live comfortably in a body, and how to find purpose in their lives. In both areas you can only transmit to them what you have realized yourself. You can say all kinds of things, but they will be just words and ideas unless they are alive within you. Touching your inner landscape and valuing your inner experiences will enhance not only your own life but the lives of your students and everyone around you.

And progressing along our own inner journey of self-discovery, we join the Upanishadic sages who dove within in pursuit of the ultimate Truth, the ultimate Reality. The *Upanishads* are experienced realities, not abstract ideas. Our modern sensibilities struggle with the idea of a subjective truth that is realized within one's own inner world and is not easily objectively verifiable.

The scientific method is an amazing and profoundly valuable asset, as it encourages us to test our hypotheses rather than just believe whatever our thoughts or emotions serve up as truth. But it has become so synonymous with materialism that we think of something as verifiable only if it can be proven in the outer, physical world. The seers of the *Upanishads* surely used the scientific method – they tested and re-tested and shared and compared their experiences, but they did not depend on material reality as the sole definer of truth and reality.

We can do the same. Within us is a world that is complex and multidimensional, populated and penetrated by beings (*devas* and *asuras* and everything in between) and forces that seek to support our self-realization or lead us astray. Not everything we find can be trusted. We need to be rigorous in our self-seeking, but not with materialism as the proof. Love is the proof, the touchstone, the guiding light that illuminates our inner darkness. Not a superficial and selfish emotion that often passes for love in our modern world – but love that is wholeness, self-giving and self-nurturing, love that is unity, truth. This is the love that is yoga.

The re-union of the Divine One and the Divine Many takes place not in some theoretical cosmic realm. It takes place here, in your body, in your life, in your mind. And the best way of discerning whether you are heading in the right direction on the path of purification is love. Your heart has an innate ability to sense love. We need to release selfishness, fear and greed in order to activate and empower this sense, but it is a natural part of our embodiment. If you are unclear whether a certain belief or behavior is serving your growth toward wholeness, look for love. Don't look for ideas about love, look for the presence of love itself as a felt experience in your heart and it will lead you always toward truth and the purity of your own being.

"Beloved, lead us from falsehood to truth, from darkness to light, and from death to immortality." The *Pavamāna* prayer is not a rejection of life, but the innate and natural cry of the separated self to be joined with All. This longing for union fuels evolution. It transforms and progressively purifies your mind, your life, and your body. The body will become a true and pure home for the soul, not by destroying it or repressing its natural desires, but by releasing the desires that serve separation and not wholeness, enmity and not love. This process is collective and inevitable; it is the sweep of evolution. We can join in the flow, or we can be carried forward while we struggle and cling to the past. The path of purification frees us to let go of all that would hold us back and become the flow toward yoga, toward the embodiment of universal love.

> "In its essence, we may think of the purification process as initiated by spiritual light and sustained by light in order to carry out the Will of the Divine. This Will moves in the direction of enabling the higher dimensions of one's being to take part in life on Earth. It allows the soul to merge with the personality in the expression of a unified and sacred life."
>
> *- GurujiMa, What is Purification, Part 1*

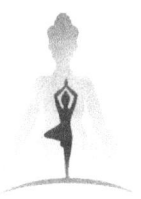

Sādhana - Spiritual Practice and Discipline

Yoga is a progressive self-discovery, and the entire Earth is on the path of yoga. I can choose to willingly participate, accelerating my own advancement on the path, or I can choose not to pay any attention. Either way, I am carried along on the current of the Earth's yoga.

In 1929, the Mother said to a few disciples:

"There are two paths of Yoga, one of tapasya (discipline), and the other of surrender. The path of tapasya is arduous. Here you rely solely upon yourself, you proceed by your own strength. You ascend and achieve according to the measure of your force. There is always the danger of falling down. And once you fall, you lie broken in the abyss and there is hardly a remedy. The other path, the path of surrender, is safe and sure. It is here, however, that the Western people find their difficulty. They have been taught to fear and avoid all that threatens their personal independence. They have imbibed with their mothers' milk the sense of individuality. And surrender means giving up all that.

"In other words, you may follow, as Ramakrishna says, either the path of the baby monkey or that of the baby cat. The baby monkey holds to its mother in order to be carried about and it must hold firm, otherwise if it loses its grip, it falls. On the other hand, the baby cat does not hold to its mother, but is held by the mother and has no fear nor responsibility; it has nothing to do but to let the mother hold it and cry 'Ma Ma!' If you take up this path of surrender fully and sincerely, there is no more danger or serious difficulty. The question is to be sincere. If you are not sincere, do not begin Yoga. If you were dealing in human affairs, then you could resort to deception; but in dealing with the Divine there is no possibility of deception anywhere."

Ramakrishna Paramahansa was a great 19th century yogi from Bengal. The words referred to by the Mother are recorded in the [Gospel of Ramakrishna Volume 1](). Ramakrishna tells a disciple that:

"It is no doubt necessary to practice spiritual discipline; but there are two kinds of aspirants. The nature of the one kind is like that of the young monkey, and the nature of the other kind is like that of the kitten. The young monkey, with great exertion, somehow clings to its mother. Likewise, there are some aspirants who think that in order to realize God they must repeat His name a certain number of times, meditate on Him for a certain period, and practice a certain amount of austerity. An aspirant of this kind makes his own efforts to catch hold of God. But the kitten, of itself, cannot cling to its mother. It lies on the ground and cries, 'Mew, mew!' It leaves everything to its mother. The mother cat sometimes puts it on a bed, sometimes on the roof behind a pile of wood. She carries the kitten in her mouth hither and thither. The kitten doesn't know how to cling to the mother. Likewise, there are some aspirants who cannot practice spiritual discipline by calculating about japa or the period of meditation. All that they do is cry to God with yearning hearts. God hears their cry and cannot keep Himself away. He reveals Himself to them."

This parable illustrates two different approaches to yoga *sādhana* (practice). In one, all the responsibility is on the *sādhaka*. I have to choose which practices to do, create time and space to do them, and make sure that I'm consistent. In the other approach, the Divine is responsible for my *sādhana*. The Mother sets the agenda, gives the practices, creates the time and space, and provides the motivation to continue. It sounds easy, but to take this second approach with sincerity, I have to actually give up the sense that I am the owner of my life, the doer of my actions. Otherwise I'll be pulling in two different directions, simultaneously toward surrender and toward agency.

For most of us, spontaneous, complete surrender to the Divine is not possible. As Sri Aurobindo wrote to a disciple, "If there is not a complete surrender, then it is not possible to adopt the baby cat attitude, — it becomes mere tamasic passivity calling itself surrender. If a complete surrender is not possible in the beginning, it follows that personal effort is necessary." And in the seminal commentary on Patañjali's Yoga Sutras, Vyāsa reminds us that it's not possible to jump from the beginning to the end without moving through stages. A child does not learn to walk in a day. "Yoga is reached through yoga. One who perseveres in yoga rejoices in yoga."

We progress by degrees, clarifying and purifying the layers of our nature until the Divine Will can flow freely through without obstruction or obfuscation. Along the way, the structure of regular, consistent practices can help. When we reserve time every day for meditation, or *asana*, or prayer, the regularity of it trains our minds and bodies to remember the state of peace and equanimity that these practices cultivate. The practices also directly support the purification process by infusing our bodies, minds and emotions with the clear light of our deeper being and helping to release impurities that have accumulated throughout this lifetime and before.

When we incarnate as humans, we do not arrive as a clean slate. We carry *karma* from previous lives, including wounds, patterned reactions, and mechanisms for coping with the brutality and seeming meaninglessness of suffering. These tendencies are called *sanskāras* in Sanskrit. They are karmic impressions created by our past choices and actions, stretching back through countless lifetimes and stored in a kind of cosmic warehouse that follows us from life to life. Almost all humans, except perhaps direct *avatars* of the Divine who have taken birth for a specific cosmic purpose, are born with *sanskāras*.

These *sanskāras* ignite mental activity in us and keep it swirling, resisting our best efforts to escape the whirlpool and achieve tranquility. They block our vision from perceiving our true nature, and like seeds, they sprout and then produce new seeds, keeping the wheel of life and death and rebirth, called *sansāra*, turning. *Sansāra* literally means a passage or migration, and it refers to the wandering, circuitous path that we take from life to life, bound by *karma*, controlled by our impulsive reactions to external circumstances.

Sanskāras are the karmic seeds that shape our core beliefs, habits and impulses. When we face a new and unexpected situation, they determine our reactions. But we always have a choice, and the practices of yoga increase the space between stimulus and response. When we become more aware of our habits and patterns of reactivity, we are more able to choose actions that flow from inspiration rather than reaction. Instead of rooting and sprouting, karmic *sanskāras* dry up and become impotent

Consistent practices grant us access to the present moment, which is where the choice exists. If someone insults me, my habitual reaction may be to shout at them, or to defend myself. But if I am fully conscious and aware in that moment, then I will notice that my reaction will not only unnecessarily increase the suffering for the other person, but for myself as well. I will realize that it will lead to the creation of new *karma* that I'll need to work out later. This awareness will allow me to choose to remain calm and equanimous, responding with clear firmness joined with compassion for whatever caused the person to insult me in the first place.

Impurities can manifest in all the layers of our being, from the most material to the most subtle. Physical impurities make our body sick, out of harmony, and unable to transmit spiritual Light. Emotional impurities create disturbances and turbulence in our emotional bodies, interfering with the depth of peace and love that are our true nature. Mental impurities affect our minds, clouding them with doubt, arrogance and confusion. The many practices of the yoga traditions address each of these layers in different ways.

Yogic *sādhana* can include practices like *asana* and bandha, *mudra*, *pranayama*, *mantra* and *japa* (repetition), visualization, *pūja* (worship), *dhyāna* (concentration), *kīrtan*, and more. *Asana, bandha,* and *mudra* work directly on the body, stretching, squeezing, massaging, and strengthening our tissues, organs, glands and nerve networks. The practices encourage the release of physical impurities and support the body's natural systems for self-regulation, digestion and elimination.

Practices like *pūja* and *kīrtan* work with our emotions, uplifting them and nurturing feelings of devotion, belonging and love. And practices like *japa* and *dhyāna* focus the mind, reducing mental chatter and distractibility. And of course the layers influence each other, so there's a non-linear relationship to how different practices affect each layer. All these practices involve minimizing the usual distractions of daily life and focusing attention. We may be focusing on the body, the breath, a specific word or phrase, an image, a ritual, or on love itself. All are a form of concentration.

Concentration strengthens patience, deepens peace, and makes it easier to see the subtle workings of the mind, emotions and body. If we want to understand ourselves, we need to be able to concentrate our attention and watch ourselves, what we do, what we think, what we believe, what we feel, and then also the consequences of our actions, behaviors, thoughts and impulses.

At the heart of yoga practice is concentration on the Divine. Ramakrishna also said:

"At Kamarpukur I have seen the women of the carpenter families selling flattened rice. Let me tell you how alert they are while doing their business. The pestle of the husking-machine that flattens the paddy constantly falls into the hole of the mortar. The woman turns the paddy in the hole with one hand and with the other holds her baby on her lap as she nurses it. In the meantime customers arrive. The machine goes on pounding the paddy, and she carries on her bargains with the customers. She says to them, 'Pay the few pennies you owe me before you take anything more.' You see, she has all these things to do at the same time — nurse the baby, turn the paddy as the pestle pounds it, take the flattened rice out of the hole, and talk to the buyers. This is called the yoga of practice. Fifteen parts of her mind out of sixteen are fixed on the pestle of the husking-machine, lest it should pound her hand. With only one part of her mind she nurses the baby and talks to the buyers. Likewise, he who leads the life of a householder should devote fifteen parts of his mind to God; otherwise he will face ruin and fall into the clutches of Death. He should perform the duties of the world with only one part of his mind."

When we concentrate on God more and more, God's presence begins to pervade our thoughts and our lives. When we call upon God to be with us over and over, we begin to notice the Divine breath on our cheek at all times. *Sādhana* awakens our capacity to feel this subtle breath as we become increasingly sensitive and aware, and it also trains us to look for it everywhere and always.

Sādhana is the commitment to yoga, the decision to create time and space for focus. Through repetition and regularity, the practice flows into the rest of the day, so that the barrier between *sādhana* and life breaks down. Then, increasingly, we are engaged with yoga all the time. There is no longer a compartment for yoga practice that remains separate from our other daily tasks, relationships, interactions, work and diversions. We live one life, more and more integrated and whole.

One reason that our lives can become fragmented when we take up a yoga practice is that we tend to do work for personal gain and to satisfy our desires. We have an underlying agenda other than the completion of the work itself. We do our yoga practices and dedicate ourselves to seeking truth, and then we go back to a way of living that doesn't resonate with that aspiration. But any work can become a *sādhana* when it is done as an offering and with the intention of letting it be a pathway for soul expression. As Sri Aurobindo wrote to a disciple, "if one can dedicate oneself through work, that is one of the most powerful means towards the self-giving which is itself the most powerful and indispensable element of the *sādhana*."

When work is done with a personal agenda it creates *karma*, consequences that ripple unseen through the fabric of the cosmos and then circle back to seek resolution. But when work is done as *sādhana*, as *seva* or service, as an offering to others, to the Earth, or to the Divine, it does not create new *karma*. It flows out from us in its purity and moves us toward freedom to realize and be our true selves.

Whatever we do can be a *sādhana*, as long as it includes concentration and a spiritual aspiration to know ourselves and the Divine. A very effective practice that can be incorporated into any task or endeavor is to concentrate your attention on your heart and imagine the Divine Mother sitting there within. This focus will gradually quiet the mind, open the heart, and invite the Mother to join in whatever work you are doing. Over time, this practice becomes natural and seamless, as simple and familiar as breathing. And as the Mother's force becomes more and more familiar within you, the sense of separateness from Her diminishes until all that you do is done for Her, with Her, and eventually by Her.

"A time will come when you will feel more and more that you are the instrument and not the worker. For first by the force of your devotion your contact with the Divine Mother will become so intimate that at all times you will have only to concentrate and to put everything into her hands to have her present guidance, her direct command or impulse, the sure indication of the thing to be done and the way to do it and the result. And afterwards you will realise that the divine Shakti not only inspires and guides, but initiates and carries out your works; all your movements are originated by her, all your powers are hers; mind, life and body are conscious and joyful instruments of her action, means for her play, moulds for her manifestation in the physical universe. There can be no more happy condition than this union and dependence; for this step carries you back beyond the borderline from the life of stress and suffering in the ignorance into the truth of your spiritual being, into its deep peace and its intense Ananda." *(from* The Mother, *by Sri Aurobindo)*

Guru: A Guide on the Path

It's often very difficult for us to know what supports we need as we transform and grow along the path of yoga. Choosing from the plethora of practices, which ones to take up and for how long and how often is daunting, and many times we just don't have the perspective to see what we need. We are too close to ourselves, too immersed in our own process to self-diagnose and prescribe treatment. We need an outsider, someone who can look at us, assess the situation, and make a recommendation. Historically, this has been the role of the yoga *guru*.

In eight-hundred CE, it wasn't possible to skip down to Barnes and Noble and purchase a *tantrik* text, and then go home and get started on your liberation. A *guru* has historically been an unequivocal necessity in yoga. During the initial flourishing of *tantra*, when the Śaiva *Siddhānta* tradition was expanding throughout India, there was a distinction between regular people going about their lives, fulfilling their social roles and performing their inherited socio-religious rituals, and *tantrikas*, who were accepted by a *guru* and initiated into the secret tradition. Generally, before seeking out a *guru*, a person would have an experience of śaktipāta, or a descent of divine energy that awakens the inner being. This śaktipāta experience could be intense, immediate, and violent, or it could evolve more gradually over time, but it essentially was an inner process of awakening that signaled the beginning of a spiritual quest, not its end.

After a śaktipāta experience, one would seek out, or perhaps synchronistically encounter, a *guru*. The guru would take on the task of supporting the integration of that experience and expanding on it, peeling away layers of delusion to reveal greater and greater degrees of truth. Because of the ego's nature, it was understood that facing oneself is not possible without a *guru's* direction, support, and care. There were rare cases in which the *guru* role was fulfilled by an inner relationship with the Divine, but this Divine Being was experienced as separate from the ego-self throughout the process of initiation, progressive integration, and liberation.

This is an area where things in the west have gotten very mixed up. We long for truth, we aspire to know ourselves and uncover our true nature. And we are surrounded by countless books, movies, podcasts, facebook posts, and every other kind of information package. Voices assail us to buy, subscribe, join, and gain what we are looking for. Simultaneously, we hear endless stories of gurus who have manipulated their position, taken advantage of their power, and victimized their community. This combination of forces compels us to seek to control our spiritual path, so we don't fall into the wrong hands. But the problem is that any real spiritual path will absolutely require a release of control. Control and liberation are diametrically opposed.

The reality is that we are not afraid of being deceived by a false guru. We are afraid of our own smallness. We are afraid that there is no Divine

Being guiding our path, and that if we fall in a hole or off a cliff, it's because we failed.

When we want something for ourselves, when the ego has manipulated our spiritual longing into a self-aggrandizing desire, we are vulnerable to manipulation by others. When we grasp for something that will make us feel bigger, better, smarter, stronger, then whoever offers us that golden chalice assumes a false power over us. But when we surrender our self, when we make an offering of the ego and its desires, then the inner light of discernment will guide us by a path that we know not. We will be carried, and even when we are engulfed by the deepest impenetrable darkness, we will move inexorably forward. The true *guru* will appear, the one whose love is pure and without need, the one whose heart is whole and has nothing to gain or lose.

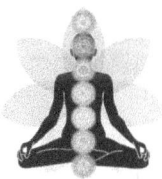

Karma, Jñana, and Bhakti

In the Bhagavad Gita, Krishna describes three approaches to liberation that have historically tended to become isolated within various lineages or schools. There are some teachers who preach a doctrine of **karma yoga** (the yoga of service), others who practice *jñāna* **yoga** (the yoga of knowledge), and others still who pursue ***bhakti* yoga** (the yoga of devotion). In a masterful way that gathers all the little strands of each path, Krishna weaves them together into a single teaching that encompasses and exceeds them all. And he also expands and clarifies each path, drawing out its nuances and defining it in a way that compliments the others rather than excluding them.

It is true that individuals tend to have a preference for one approach over the others, and there is nothing wrong with that. We each have our own *svabhāva*, our own unique nature. But when we say "I'm a *bhakta*," or "I'm not a *bhakta*, I'm a *jñāni*," we do run the risk of creating an unnecessary exclusivity and cutting ourselves off from an important aspect of ourselves. Just like the three *gūnas* exist in different proportions in every aspect of existence, the three paths of yoga exist in different proportions in all of us, and this is not static. One path may predominate for a time, giving way to the emergence of another. I may be inclined for a while toward textual study and mental inquiry in the search for myself, and then later the flame of devotion may arise within.

Inevitably, as we move forward along a path of self-discovery, we will be inclined to explore different approaches to truth. If we maintain a fixed idea that one approach is ours for all time, then we will limit the soul's natural movement to freely explore all dimensions of our inner landscape. And, the better I know God, the more I will love God, and the more I love God the more I will come to know God. And as I offer the fruits of my work in the world to God, my understanding and love will inevitably deepen. These three paths ultimately unite, as they all lead in the same direction.

Karma Yoga

Karma yoga is the practice of offering one's work to the Divine. In the Bhagavad Gita, Krishna puts it in terms of the fruits of our actions. We generally act with an eye to reaping rewards. We work a job in order to get paid, plan a vacation in order to relax and enjoy, donate to charity in order to feel generous and helpful.

In the Devīmahatmya, a yogi teaches a king and a merchant about karma yoga with a metaphor about birds. He says that birds, even though they feel the pangs of hunger, give their scarce food to their young without any thought or expectation of reciprocation. People on the other hand have all kinds of expectations and attachments with regard to their children. These expectations and attachments often lead to frustration, resentment, disappointment and suffering. But when we just offer ourselves selflessly, without attachment or expectation or entitlement, just do the work given to us with a humble generosity of spirit, even when the work is hard and involves sacrifice, we experience freedom and grace.

When we think of ourselves as the "doer" who decides and plans and executes the activities of our life, then we tend to feel entitled to the fruits of our actions and efforts. But Krishna explains that we are not really the "doer" at all. Most of what we do is the result of habits, fears, old karmic patterns, and reactions to circumstances. We are pushed and pulled by forces of nature inside and outside of ourselves. The only way to be free of this dynamic is to discover our inner nature, which is born of and one with the Divine Being and offer ourselves entirely to that.

Karma yoga is the practice and process of offering ourselves by offering our work, our efforts, our plans, and the results and rewards of our work to the Divine. When I practice, I naturally begin to experience myself as in relationship with all of life. My perspective shifts from being overly focused on I, me, and mine to experiencing myself as belonging to all, and this experience is both deeply satisfying and fundamentally true. I begin to know that I am never alone, never isolated, and always in relationship.

As we come to know the nature of reality, when we have inquired into and explored the layers and phenomena of existence and come to understand the nature of causation, the reality of *karma*, and the delusion of what we normally consider free will, then our actions do not bind us: *"As a fire kindled turns to ashes its fuel, O Arjuna, so the fire of knowledge turns all works to ashes." (Bhagavad Gita 4.37)*

When we act from within ego-created delusion, thinking that we are an individual self that acts upon an inert and separate world, then we are unwittingly bound by the invisible consequences of our actions. Instead our actions can arise from an enlightened alignment with the true Self, our soul's personality, called *purusha* in the yoga traditions. The *purusha* is inherently joined with all and thus always seeks to serve all. When we act from this place, our actions facilitate liberation for ourselves and others.

Krishna explains to Arjuna that he has two different aspects: a lower aspect that manifests as *prakriti*, and a higher aspect that is free and independent of *prakriti*:

"Earth, water, fire, air, ether, sense-mind, ego, and reasoning mind – this is my eightfold nature. This is the lower. Know too, O mighty-armed, my other Nature which is different from this, the Supreme which becomes the individual soul and by which this world is upheld. Know this to be the womb of all beings. I am the birth of the whole world and also its dissolution." (7.4, 5, 6)

Jñana Yoga

Jñana yoga is the practice of seeking truth through knowledge. In the yoga traditions, often this seeking takes the form of discrimination. We inquire into the nature of reality and the nature of self, gradually peeling away layers and unveiling deeper and deeper truths. The great 20th century yogi Ramana Maharshi simplified and condensed the path of jñana yoga into a single question: "Who am I?"

Ramana encouraged his disciples to ask this question incessantly, and to constantly notice all the things that we tend to consider "me" but actually are not. Am I my job? Am I my clothes? Am I my body, my thoughts, my preferences, my beliefs? Am I the ideas that others have about me? Who am I really? Where is this elusive I?

Eventually, this inquiry leads to a single realization: I am. Not "I think, therefore I am" as proclaimed by the western thinker Descartes. Just "I am". And that "I am" is not an isolated, fragmented sense of identity living in a bubble. It reverberates throughout the cosmos. It lives within me and within the Earth, in the sun and the stars, and in the heart of every being. Knowing myself, I know all, and I know The All that is God.

Jñana yoga is essentially a purification of understanding, a clearing out of false beliefs and identifications that prevent us from knowing who we are. We are born into a state of confusion and delusion. We live in a world that reinforces that confusion, encouraging us to identify as our personality and our ideas, to experience life through our thoughts. Identifying and releasing the delusion is a huge task because it's a matter of identity. How can I let go of myself?

The path is twofold. On the one hand, we have to separate from the false "I" that commands our attention. We have to progressively untangle from the personality so that it becomes like a shirt that can be taken on or off, but does not define us. On the other hand we have to fix our attention on the One, the Infinite, the Eternal Being. By concentrating on the One, the experience of union gradually, organically grows. It takes the place of our habitual experience of the self as separate and isolated. We slowly realize the truth of our essential nature as a ray of that Light, a wave inseparable from the ocean of God.

Jñana yoga involves both contemplation and concentration. Contemplation is an iterative process, one through which we consider thoughts and ideas, ours and those of others. We can sit quietly and observe our thoughts, noting their patterns, the way one thought needs to another, stretching and twisting and sometimes crossing over unseen from fact to fiction. And we can read the teachings and ideas presented by yogis throughout time.

There are endless profound spiritual texts from the yoga tradition that invite contemplation and transmit wisdom. But sitting with these texts, absorbing them and letting them wash over us, we are influenced by their light. Our minds are transformed and drawn into deeper and deeper layers of reality. In his commentary on Patañjali's Yoga Sūtras, Vyāsa defines *svadhyāya* as reading spiritual texts. The meaning of the word is closer to self study, but this definition reveals that study of spiritual texts is really a study of ourselves.

Concentration is focused awareness. We gather our consciousness and direct it onto a single object, working intentionally to stay there. We ignore and avoid the discursive thought process, wandering through the mind from one place to the next. We continually bring ourselves back to the object of focus, training our attention to stay put, disempowering the habit of wandering off.

When we concentrate on anything, a candle flame, a mantra, our breath, or a vision of the Divine Mother in our heart, we come home to our self. Everything in this vast, complex cosmos is made of the same stuff. Under all the difference is sameness, belonging, unity. And eventually concentration on anything opens the door to that layer of oneness. The individuality of the object breaks down and we find ourselves staring into the depth of our own soul.

Bhakti Yoga

Ramana Maharshi is known as a great *jñana* yogi whose teachers pointed incessantly toward the Self that underlies all selves. But he was also a lover of God, and he wrote and recited beautiful songs and poetry to Śiva. He realized that the substance that holds together the Earth and keeps the planets revolving around the sun and the heart beating and the rivers flowing is not some mechanical abstraction. It is love.

Truly, when we come to know the Divine One, then we cannot help but fall to our knees in devotion. And when we love the Supreme Being with all our heart, then we cannot help but come to know and understand That One. Whichever path we begin upon, we will eventually find the other, for they inevitably join.

> "At the end of many births, the seeker of knowledge attains to Me and sees that Vasudeva, the omnipresent Being, is all that is."
> *(Bhagavad Gita 7.19)*

The natural relationship of a part to its whole is devotion, reverence, and love. A fruit naturally worships the tree from which it grows, a tree loves the forest that nourishes it, and a forest resonates with gratitude and bhakti for the Earth. God is our source, and the whole that comprises all Our innate honoring of the Divine Beloved is not something that we fabricate or contrive. We discover it by removing the layers of false beliefs, fear, and coping mechanisms that we have developed to deal with the experience of separation.

When we incarnated as humans on Earth, we left the experience of infinite oneness with the source of our being; we left the experience of being upheld and supported and surrounded by love. That reality is still within us, but it's buried, and we have turned to behaviors that seem to approximate that experience of comfort and belonging, but in reality don't provide true satisfaction. These behaviors become addictions to relationships, to control, to distraction, to getting high on adrenaline, drugs and drama. Releasing these coping mechanisms and seeking for something invisible requires courage, perseverance and faith.

Tirumular was one of the sixty-three Tamil *Nayanars*. The word literally means "hounds of *Śiva*", and speaks to their unflagging devotion to their master. The *Nayanars* were powerful embodiments of Śiva bhakti in Tamil Nadu during the first millennium CE, and remain inspirational figures throughout the region today. These poet/singer saints gave themselves to devotion and expounded a doctrine of loving surrender to Śiva as a path to liberation. They found divine bliss, and sought to share it with the world: "May this world share the bliss that I have had" (*Thirumanthiram*).

The legend goes that a yogi named Sundarar was living on Mount Kailash in the Himalayas. On a journey south, he noticed a herd of cows gathered around the body of their cowherd, Mulan, and crying miserably. Out of compassion for the cows, Sundarar left his own body and entered that of Mulan, who immediately came to life. Sundarar, in the body of Mulan, took the cows home and then came back for his own body, which had disappeared, having been stolen by Śiva himself. The yogi/cowherd sat beneath a peepal tree and entered a deep meditative state. Eventually he came to be known by the local people as Tirumular (holy Mulan), and they would sit and wait for him to periodically emerge from Samādhi and utter a few verses, which they recorded. In all they took down three-thousand verses, which form the *Thirumanthiram*.

Thirumanthiram is the earliest known of the Tamil *tantrik* texts. It was composed in poetic meter and covers a wide range of topics, including metaphysics, mantras and yantras, references to Patañjali's 8-limbed yoga, and the means to attain *kaya siddhi*, or a perfected and immortal body. But its central message is *Anbe* Śivam: Love is Śiva. Śiva is the source and inner being of everything – He did not create the universe as something apart from Himself; He became the universe, or more appropriately, He is constantly becoming the universe. And Love is Śiva, the inner self of all.

"The ignorant rant that Love and Śiva are two,
They know not that Love alone is Śiva
When we learn that Love and Śiva are the same
Love as Śiva, they ever remain…

…Worship the Lord with heart melted in love;
When we direct our love to God, He too approaches us with love…

…Offer the flower of 'you' at the feet of 'He';
Then no more will you speak of 'you' and 'He'."
– *Thirumanthiram 270, 275 and 1607*

Bhakti yoga does the same thing with our emotions that jñana yoga does with our minds. It seeks the purity that underlies all the layers of confusion. And just as great *jñana* teachings have been gathered into texts over thousands of years, inviting seekers to read and contemplate, great bhakti teachings have been recorded in texts, songs and poetry. A human heart's natural state is to be immersed in love for God. These texts, songs and poetry capture that raptured state of love and bring it to life.

The contemplations and concentrations of jñana yoga can often lead to an experience of absence (the word *nirvāna* means to be blown out like a candle flame). We look at the various things that we habitually identify as self and realize that they are false identifications, leaving us with a sense that nothing is actually real. I am not this, nor am I this. As the Brihadaranyaka Upanishad says, *neti neti*. Bhakti contemplations and practices, on the other hand, lead to an experience of fullness. Singing to God, praying to God, contemplating the beauty and majesty of God all lead to a deepening of the experience that God Is. And when I realize further that God is everything, even me, then I find that myself is not empty at all, but eternally full.

This dynamic between fullness and emptiness is contained in the yogic understanding that there exists a *nirguna brahman*, divinity without qualities or attributes, a primordial nothingness out of which all creation comes, and a *saguna brahman*, divinity with attributes, the radiant totality of the manifest divine. In the Bhagavad Gīta, Krishna tells Arjuna that he encompasses both saguna and nirguna. As the *purushottama*, the ultimate personality, he embraces both the nonexistent and all of existence. He declares that these two apparent opposites are in fact two sides of one coin. And that coin is Krishna himself.

What can we do in the face of that impossibly eternal radiant being other than worship? How can we respond other than with singing and praise? The natural upwelling of our hearts when we see or hear the Divine, when we feel the Holy Breath upon our cheek, is reverence and rejoicing. God exists, and all our fears are held within the divine embrace. God is, and God is everything, and everything is love.

Synthesis

This interwoven yoga of service, knowledge and devotion is Krishna's offering to Arjuna, and to the world. He invites us to find and experience all the dimensions of our relationship with the Divine, to let them flow into each other and expand each other. And when we join heart, mind and hands, unifying our life in a single direction, we are sure to arrive at our destination.

Each of us is one and together we are One. The universal light of creation flows through every created being, and yoga is the path that leads to rediscovering this light within us. We live fragmented lives, putting on different personalities based on our surroundings and who we are trying to impress, prioritizing different aspects of ourselves depending on what we are trying to achieve or avoid. But really we are one radiant flame, and our lives are meant to reflect that flame and shine it in every direction. Every true path of yoga leads in this direction, whether it be through work, thought or love.

"Devoting all thyself to Me, giving up in thy conscious mind all thy actions into Me, resorting to Yoga of the will and intelligence, be always one in heart and consciousness with Me. By aligning your heart and consciousness with Me at all times, by My grace you will pass safely through all difficult and perilous passages." *(Bhagavad Gītā 18.57, 58)*

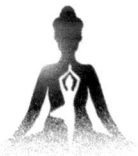

All Life Is Yoga: The Path of Karma and The Path of Dharma

Karma

Karma is one of those yoga words that has made its way into the modern English lexicon. It has mixed with western spiritual ideas and taken on the sense of divine justice, almost retribution, a balancing of the scales so that those who act badly get a taste of their own medicine. What has been lost is the context of a soul on a learning journey that encompasses many lifetimes and always trends toward wholeness.

In the yoga traditions, karma is understood to be a law or a force like gravity. It is universally applicable and organizes the universe by pulling beings toward truth. But it's not isolated to one lifetime. Karma accrued in one life can unfold through experiences and circumstances in another, even though the person may not remember anything about the source of the karma. And it's not just about justice or punishment. It's also about healing.

Let's say that I died from drowning in a previous life. The trauma from this experience would carry forward into future lifetimes. The memories would lay unconscious within my field of being and become embodied when I took birth. Innate preferences, habits, fears and attractions would travel into this life from the past and be taken for granted as "me". I may have an inexplicable fear of water, or of boats, or of choking. These primary fears, depending on how people around us respond to them when we're young, could be covered over by additional layers of psychological patterns, like generalized anxiety, obsessive compulsive tendencies, or a tendency toward aggression when challenged.

This is not all. The force of karma acts not just through inner experience, but shapes external life events as well, and it's oriented toward healing and growing toward wholeness. The science of astrology is essentially a way of understanding karmic influences and how they unfold within a life. So in the case of a prior life that ended with drowning, the force of karma would create life circumstances that enable healing of the trauma and release of the false layers of personality. The innate imbalance would be illuminated and challenged. Karma does not operate through force or negate our free will. It creates opportunities, and then it's up to us to choose them.

The hardest thing about all this is that it has to do with identity. If who I experience myself to be, what I take for granted as "me" is constructed of experiences that predate my current birth, then it's harder to see them as external and easier to take them for granted. The sense of my self feels solid and substantial, but it's actually based on a delusion.

The path of yoga involves an intentional decision to transcend this delusion. Sri Aurobindo calls the part of us that travels through lifetimes, learning and growing, the psychic being. He distinguishes this from the soul, that fundamental spark of divine flame that was created by God "in the beginning". In order to know my soul, I must first shift from thinking of my personality as my self and realize the deeper layer of my psychic being. The journey of the psychic being then reveals the destination, which is also the origin: the soul.

Challenging the delusion of self can be very destabilizing, especially if we don't have another ground to stand on. But if I have experienced my psychic being or my soul essence, then I have a sense that if I step away from identification with my ego self, I'm not just in free fall. I'm stepping into something much wider and vaster, something unharmable, eternal, free and beautiful.

Sri Aurobindo and GurujiMa both teach that this process of evolution toward wholeness is not something that happens to individuals in isolation. We are all evolving together. The Earth herself is a being and she is evolving, growing toward wholeness. There is a universal harmony that emerges when individuals sing their true note, aligned with their soul self. The manifestation of this harmony on Earth is the purpose for Earth's existence. That's why she was created: to nurture and channel this glorious harmony of Truth, singing Her song, our song into the cosmos.

I can't change you or force you to evolve more quickly, but I can attend to my own path of yoga and seek to sing my own true song, the song of my soul. When I do, my song resonates vibrationally and invites harmony. It invites you to sing not the same note or song as me, but your own true note, the one that compliments and amplifies mine, as mine does to yours.

Dharma

The force of karma works hidden from view, influencing much of human activity and behavior. Mostly we are reactive, being driven by habits, preferences, fears and desires that we don't see. We drive into conflicts and consequences and feel frustrated and out of control. We get angry to help ourselves feel less helpless. But there is an alternative. When we shift from the path of karma to the path of dharma, we stop being reactively pushed and pulled by unseen forces.

The path of dharma is the path of yoga. It is the path of service to the wholeness of which we are part. It is the path of love for ourselves and love for all creation. The path of dharma is the decision to live with purpose and to unify our life around that purpose. Instead of living to gain and hoarding or protecting the fruits of our labor, we live to give and serve. We live to be in harmony with the force of love and goodness that is the light of creation.

Often as we awaken spiritually, it happens in compartments. We begin to understand spiritual ideas and read spiritual books. We meditate and engage in other yoga practices, and carve out some time in our lives for pursuing spirituality. But the path of dharma is holistic, and its nature is to pull more and more of the fragments of our lives into its orbit. Spiritual ideas start to seem abstract, or in conflict with the basic daily decisions that define our lives. This conflict calls for resolution. Sometimes it leads us to feel cynical or disillusioned, ready to forget about spiritual ideals that we aren't able to embody, and that we don't see others manifesting.

Retreating into cynicism can work for a time, but eventually the desire to know ourselves resurfaces. It returns because it is the fundamental force of nature. When the Divine One spun Herself into a million trillion individualities, She embedded the inclination toward reunification into every one. She embedded a homing mechanism into the fabric of our being, and it will never let up. It might feel like dissatisfaction, boredom, emptiness, frustration, irritability, despair, or anxiety. These experiences conceal their deeper source: the longing to know and be the truth of our being.

Living within the web of karma, we ask "how can I get my needs met?" We struggle and strive to make ends meet and please people and to find time for me. We work and watch our savings and plan for vacations and keep track of who owes us a favor or who we are indebted to. We move through life entranced by habits, held in recurring patterns of thought and behavior.

When we shift into alignment with dharma, we say "I am the love that heals the world." We open and offer ourselves to life without worrying about what the reward will be. We look around us with awe at the constantly unfolding miracle, and wonder what we can contribute to it. Habits lose their gravity and thoughts and behaviors become free expressions of soul. We sing the unique song that we were born to sing.

The path of dharma takes us toward the truth of our being. When we decide to walk upon it, we intend to give ourselves to this great awakening and offer our whole lives in service to it. We open to guidance from the Divine Beloved, who constantly whispers in our ear if we take the time to listen. We structure our lives around this guidance, allowing big and small decisions to flow from deeper and deeper within us. Instead of calculating the potential losses and gains, adding up the pros and cons of a decision to take a job or buy a car or take a trip or go for a walk or apply to a college or take a workshop or cook a specific meal, we tune in to the wordless flow of truth that we are beneath all the thoughts and words. We seek to feel the current of divine life moving through us and allow it to touch all that we do.

In this way, a whole life becomes yoga. Yoga is no longer a practice or a mantra, a lifestyle or a job. It is not a class we attend or something we do. Yoga is everything we think, do, say, believe, eat, and breathe. It is our very being at every moment. And when all of life becomes yoga, then we open the door to a life divine, not in some far away heaven beyond the clouds, but here on this sacred Earth.

International Publications

Auroville Architecture
by Franz Fassbender

Auroville Form Style and Design
by Franz Fassbender

Landscapes and Gardens of Auroville
by Franz Fassbender

Inauguration of Auroville
by Franz Fassbender

Auroville in a Nutshell
by Tim Wrey

Death doesn't exist
The Mother on Death, Sri Aurobindo on Rebirth *Compiled*
by Franz Fassbender

Divine Love
Compiled by Franz Fassbender

Five Dream
by Sri Aurobindo

Vision
Compiled by Franz Fassbender

Passage to More than India
by Dick Batstone

The Mother on Japan
Compiled by Franz Fassbender

Children of Change: A Spiritual Pilgrimage
by Amrit (Howard Shoji Iriyama)

Memories of Auroville - told by early Aurovilians
by Janet Feran

The Journeying Years
by Dianna Bowler

Auroville Reflected
by Bindu Mohanty

Finding the Psychic Being
by Loretta Shartsis

The Teachings of Flowers
The Life and Work of the Mother of the Sri Aurobindo Ashram *by Loretta Shartsis*

The Supramental Transformation
by Loretta Shartsis

The Mother's Yoga - 1956-1973 (English & French)
Vol. 1, 1956-1967 & Vol. 2, 1968-1973
by Loretta Shartsis

Antithesis of Yoga
by Jocelyn Janaka

Bougainvilleas PROTECTION
by Narad (Richard Eggenberger), Nilisha Mehta

Crossroad The New Humanity
by Paulette Hadnagy

Die Praxis Des Integralen Yoga
By M. P. Pandit

The Way of the Sunlit Path
William Sullivan

Wildlife great and small of India's Coromandel
by Tim Wrey

A New Education With A Soul
by Marguerite Smithwhite

Featured Titles

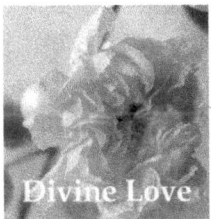

Divine Love

The texts presented in this book are selected from the Mother and Sri Aurobindo.

"Awakened to the meaning of my heart. That to feel love and oneness is to live. And this the magic of our golden change, is all the truth I know or seek, O sage."

Sri Aurobindo, Savitri, Book XII, Epilog

A Vision by the Mother

On 28th May 1958, the Mother recounted a vision she once had of a wonderful Being of Love and Consciousness, emanated from the Supreme Origin and projected directly into the Inconscient so that the creation would gradually awaken to the Supramental Consciousness. The Mother's account of this vision was brought out a first time in November 1906, in the Revue Cosmique, a monthly review published in Paris.

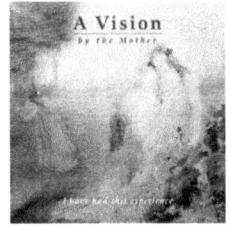

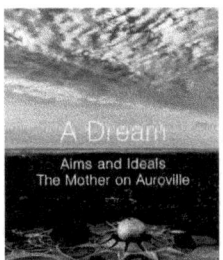

A Dream – Aims and Ideals of Auroville
the Mother on Auroville

50 years of Auroville from 28.02.1968 - 28.02.2018

Today, information about Auroville is abundant. Many people try to make meaning out of Auroville – about its conception, to what direction should we grow towards, and, what are we doing here?

But what was Mother's original Dream and what was her Vision for Auroville back then?

Matrimandir Talks by the Mother

This book presents most of Mother's Matrimandir talks, including how she conceived the idea for this special concentration and meditation building in Auroville.

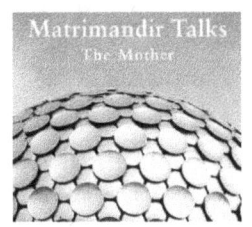

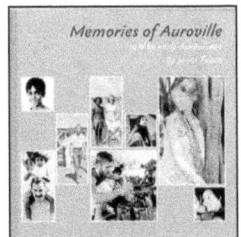

Memories of Auroville - Told by early Aurovilians

Memories of Auroville is a book about the very early days of Auroville based on interviews made in 1997 with Aurovilians who lived here between 1968 and 1973. The interviews presented in this book are part of a history program for newcomers that I had created with my friend, Philip Melville in 1997. The plan was to divide Auroville's history into different eras and then interview Aurovilians according to their area of knowledge. Our first section would cover the years from 1968 till 1973 when the Mother was still in her physical body.

The Way of the Sunlit Path

May The Way of the Sunlit Path be a convenient guide for activating this ancient truth as a support for a Conscious Evolution.
May it illumine the transformation offered to us in the Integral Yoga.

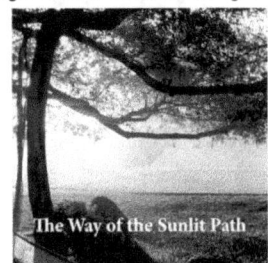

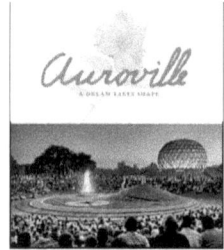

A Dream Takes Shape (in English, French, Hindi)

A comprehensive brochure on the international township of Auroville in, ranging from its Charter and "Why Auroville?" to the plan of the township, the central Matrimandir, the national pavilions and residences, to working groups, the economy, making visits, how to join, its relationship to the Sri Aurobindo Ashram, and its key role in the future of the world. This brochure endeavours to highlight how The Mother envisioned Auroville from its inception, some of the major achievements realised over the years, and some of the difficulties currently faced in implementing the guidelines which she gave.

Mother on Japan

I had everything to learn in Japan. For four years, from an artistic point of view, I lived from wonder to wonder. And everything in this city, in this country, from beginning to end, gives you the impression of impermanence, of the unexpected, the exceptional... ...everything in this city, in this country, from beginning to end, gives you the impression of impermanence, of the unexpected, the exceptional. You always come to things you did not expect; you want to find them again and they are lost – they have made something else which is equally charming.

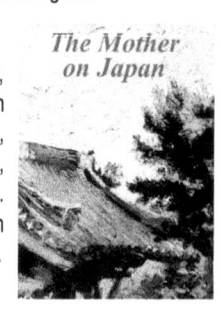

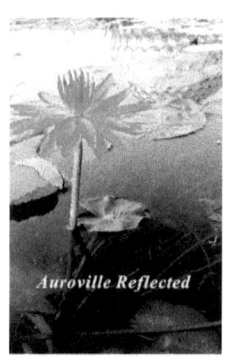

Auroville Reflected

On 28 February 1968, on an impoverished plateau on the Coromandel Coast of South India, about 4,000 people from around the world gathered for a most unusual inauguration. Handfuls of soil from the countries of the world were mixed together as a symbol of human unity. Why did Indira Gandhi, the erstwhile Prime Minister of India, support this development for "a city the earth needs?" Why did UNESCO endorse this project? Why does the Dalai Lama continue to be involved in the project? What led anthropologist Margaret Mead to insist that records must be kept of its progress? Why did both historian William Irwin Thompson and United Nations representative Robert Muller note that this social experiment may be a breakthrough for humanity even as critics commented, "it is an impossible dream"?

A House For the Third Millennium
Essays on Matrimandir

Nightwatch at the Matrimandir...
A cosmic spectacle; the black expanse above, the big black crater of Matrimandir's excavation carved deep into the soil. The four pillars - two of which are completed and the other two nearing completion - are four huge ships coming together from the four corners of the earth to meet at this pro propitious spot...

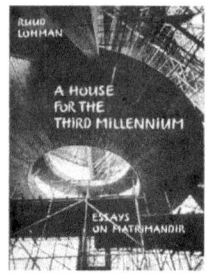

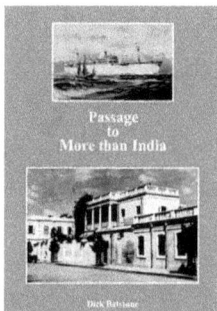

Passage to More than India

This book is a voyage of discovery. In 1959 the author, Dick Batstone, a classically educated bookseller in England, with a Christian background, comes across a life of the great Indian polymath Sri Aurobindo, though a series of apparently fortuitous circumstances. A meeting in Durham, England, leads him to a determination to get to the Sri Aurobindo Ashram in Pondicherry, a former French territory south of Madras.

www.ingramcontent.com/pod-product-compliance
Lightning Source LLC
LaVergne TN
LVHW021053100526
838202LV00083B/5842